Phyllis Langton has had as illustrious a career as anyone in academia, but she has taken infinite pains now to write a different kind of book. Her story of her husband's life with and death from ALS (Lou Gehrig's disease) yields many a valuable lesson, but this lesson above all: that dying, whatever its pains, can be both a negative and a positive experience. Here love and mortality, laughter and sorrow are all but inseparable, and their inseparability may help lessen a reader's fear of death and dying. Anyone who enjoys a deeply moving story will want to read this wondrous, indispensable book, and anybody who faces adversity, that is to say everybody, will need to read it.

Jeffery Paine—author of *Father India, Re-enchantment, Adventures with the Buddha*, and *Tales of Wonder* (with Huston Smith). Judge for the Pulitzer Prize and former vice-president of the National Book Critics Circle.

Like many others, I've not been comfortable with the subject of death—the death of my loved ones or myself. How lucky we humans are to have Phyllis Langton's story as part of our lives. This moving book has allowed me to look death in the eye, and even find a way to laugh about it. Langton shows us that deep love and laughter make the sorrow and loss bearable, paving the way for this ultimate journey and beyond. . . .

Jill Breckenridge—author of *The Gravity of Flesh* and *Miss Priss and the Con Man.*

I couldn't put *Last Flight Out* down. I wanted it to go on so I could learn more about Phyllis and George and their story about facing ALS together. George had a terminal disease and he and Phyllis chose to live and love to the fullest! What an incredible message to read especially with a disease that takes and takes.

Sharon J. Matland, R.N., M.B.A.—Vice-President of Patient Services, ALS Association

Who would have thought that disease can be a page-turner? But Phyllis Langton's bittersweet memoir of her fighter-pilot husband's last years shows that a good marriage can be as joyous in sickness as it is in health. *Last Flight Out* is a vivid, sparkling story about facing death with grace and high spirits.

Mark Weston—author of *Giants of Japan* and *Prophets and Princes: Saudi Arabia From Muhammad to the Present.*

Last Flight Out really touched my heart. As the hospice physician who cared for George, I found the description of the denial of his symptoms extremely compelling and riveting and it taught me to appreciate more deeply the psychological defenses which patients use to protect themselves against the perception of their own vulnerabilities. In addition, this memoir reminds all who read it of the paramount need to honor and respect a patient's wishes to control the conditions of care and medical treatment. George achieved a wonderful peace of mind as his disease relentlessly progressed. Everyone should be so fortunate to have such a resourceful and loving advocate for their partner.

Dr. Henry Willner—Hospice Physician and Palliative Care Consultant, Capital Hospice.

George Thomas's reaction to a diagnosis of ALS reminded me of that moment in my own life. Each of us then learned, at last, what was happening to us. Both of us now had to figure out how we were going to live the rest of our lives. Phyllis Langton has gifted us with this testimony to the way that she and George lived their answer.

On the surface this book is about Phyllis, George and ALS. As the chapters unfold we feel what it is like to live with a progressive disease. However, in words permeated with compassion, Phyllis is doing more than remembering. She is inviting us to find ourselves in her story. Like George I have ALS. Like George I'm surrounded by the love of my wife and a community of friends. We all must learn to accommodate ourselves each day to life in a body that is less able than it was yesterday. In the midst of our diverse journeys we are invited to realize the love that surrounds us and to compassionately care for others. In the end we are reminded that it is faith, hope and love that sustain us. This book had to be written. It is yearning for you to read it.

Rev. Dr. John W. Mingus, Sr.—*Retired after 37 years as an ordained minister of the United Church of Christ, now living richly with ALS in Venice, FL with his wife and two young sons.*

In my 28 years as a healthcare chaplain I have observed the journey toward death Phyllis Langton portrays in *Last Flight Out*. But I am a professional who only sees those brief moments I am at the hospital or nursing home bedside or visiting in someone's home. Langton invites us into her life with her husband George as he moves through increasing disability to his final breaths. It is moving and, in my view, honest. The prospect of a certain death is only one of the great losses Phyllis and George experienced. George is able to experience the death of his own choosing through Phyllis' commitment to honor his wishes. They live fully while he is dying. Everyone's course toward death is different but Langton's story has lessons for all of us. Enjoy the humor, find your own rituals, enlist friends and professionals to help, grieve the losses (and they are many), honor each other, and learn to let go.

Chaplain Hank Dunn—author of *Hard Choices for Loving People*.

The ALS community of patients and caregivers was not one Phyllis Langton and her late husband, George, chose to join, but the insidious disease took up residence with them during the last three years of their remarkable marriage. In *Last Flight Out* Langton does more than relate the details of her fighter pilot husband's battle with illness; she shares a transforming experience with such compelling grace and fierce love that the reader is also transformed. This is a book that will initiate conversations on illness, on marriage, on love, and certainly on the importance of people coming together to support and celebrate a life. Langton's profound memoir reminds us that as long we we are willing to share our life stories, we are never alone.

Kerry Langan—author of *Only Beautiful & Other Stories*

LAST FLIGHT OUT
Living, Loving & Leaving

BOOKS FROM WISING UP PRESS

WISING UP ANTHOLOGIES

Illness & Grace, Terror & Transformation

Families: The Frontline of Pluralism

Love After 70

Double Lives, Reinvention & Those We Leave Behind

View from the Bed: View from the Bedside

*Shifting Balance Sheets: Women's Stories of Naturalized
Citizenship & Cultural Attachment*

WISING UP PRESS COLLECTIVE

Only Beautiful & Other Stories
Kerry Langan

Keys to the Kingdom: Reflections on Music and the Mind
Kathleen L. Housley

A Hymn that Meanders
Maria Nazos

The Sanctity of the Moment: Poems from Four Decades
Heather Tosteson

LAST FLIGHT OUT
Living, Loving & Leaving

PHYLLIS A. LANGTON

Wising Up Press Collective
Wising Up Press
Decatur, Georgia

Wising Up Press
P.O. Box 2122
Decatur, GA 30031-2122
www.universaltable.org

While some names have been changed to protect identity, all characters are real and intact. No attempt was made to verify the facts my husband shared about his life before we met. What is important for this book is how he experienced his life.

Catalogue-in-Publication data is on file with the Library of Congress.
LCCN: 2011929262

Wising Up ISBN: 978-0-9827262-2-8

For Gentleman George

Letting me care for you during this entire journey was your final gift to me. By accepting my love and care you helped ease the pain of my grief in a way that only you could do. I hear you speak as I write.

TABLE OF CONTENTS

PART THREE: NOVEMBER 2002—MARCH 2003

PROLOGUE

The test of a first-rate intelligence is the ability to hold two opposed ideas in the mind at the same time, and still retain the ability to function.
                                        —F. Scott Fitzgerald

Death hung in the air that day. On September 11, 2001, I drove my husband, George, to our brand new four-story townhouse in McLean, Virginia, twenty miles from the Pentagon. Terrorists had flown airplanes that morning into the World Trade Center in New York City and the Pentagon killing thousands of innocent people.

As an Air Force officer, George's career had been defined in many ways by his assignments to the Pentagon, the last time in the late 1960's, before leaving for Vietnam. He had told me that people who worked there viewed it as America's iron fortress. As a fighter pilot, he was deeply moved by the attack.

Holding the hand-railing tightly, George walked in the front door of our townhouse with a soft smile and little assistance. After we explored the first floor, I heard him sigh, and saw his chest heave as his face turned gray.

He took my arm and said, "Where's our elevator? Let's look at the other floors."

His legs trembled as he grasped the elevator side rails.

"When I die and leave this house," he said, "I want to ride down in this elevator standing tall. An old fighter pilot of three wars can't leave his loved ones and his world feet first. I want to complete my mission with honor and dignity. I want to leave my home the way I came in, standing on my feet. Can you manage that, Phyllis?"

"Yes," I said quickly, with no idea how I would manage his request.

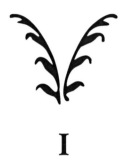

I

OCTOBER 2000—OCTOBER 2001

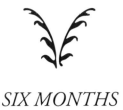

SIX MONTHS

"I know what's going to be on my death certificate. That's more than you can say."

On Wednesday morning, eleven months earlier—October 11, 2000—the neurologist, Dr. Noble, entered the waiting room that faintly smelled of Pine-Sol and human traffic. He resembled my husband, George, in many ways: medium height and build, the same full-bodied gray hair, and wearing the same style of rimless glasses over his sapphire blue eyes—eyes the color of George's. I liked him right away.

"Mr. Thomas?" he said, smiling as he introduced himself to us. His handshake felt firm, but not aggressive. George had difficulty extending his hand, and I suspected the doctor noted this. I held George's arm as we walked to the doctor's office. Out of the corner of my eye, I noticed Dr. Noble watching George walk.

As we sat in his office, looking through floor-length windows with views of the fiery red fall colors of the large maple trees, Dr. Noble told us that the reports from the referring doctors had not been sent. He had talked on the phone with one of the doctors to get his interpretations of some of the tests. "I would like to repeat some of the EMG tests to measure the strength of a few of your arm and leg muscles to confirm for myself what is going on," Dr. Noble added.

"I've had all these tests and now you want more?" George grumbled. "These tests wear me out. I'm too tired to have any more needles stuck in my muscles."

"I'm sorry," the doctor replied. "I can understand why you're upset. I just need to test two or three muscles to know whether these muscle twitches in your face and hands are a result of misfiring of the nerve cells."

Dr. Noble added, "I won't repeat the entire test. I need to review the original films from your MRI tests, and readings from the EMGs and interpret what I see, independent of what others have done."

George's head jerked up. "Thank you for explaining this to me. I've been told very little about what is being done and why. How long will your test take?"

"Not very long. I'd like to test two muscles in your arms and legs today. Given the potential gravity of any diagnosis, we need to be as sure as possible before we begin to talk about treatment and any other options."

While they went to the examining room, I found the ladies' room, sat on the toilet, and wept. *Where were the reports?* This meant another delay in knowing what was happening to him, another painful trip to a doctor's office, more tests. After washing my hands, I gripped the counter, practiced my meditation, and counted to fifty to keep from screaming.

Finally composed, I pressured the receptionist to give us another appointment two days later, on Friday. I said that I would get all the reports and drop them by that office the next morning. When I wrote down the date, I realized it would be Friday the 13th. As children, we had lived in a time when Friday the 13th was a scary day, and you didn't walk under ladders, or let black cats run in front of you. If you did, you would have bad luck all day.

We arrived at Dr. Noble's office for the final interpretation of all the tests. He told George he'd like to check him again in the examining room, while I waited in the doctor's office.

After he completed his exam and George was dressing, Dr. Noble showed me George's MRI films on the X-ray viewer on the wall. "The cervical MRI showed minimal degenerative disc change without any narrowing or bulging. It wasn't conclusive," he said.

"Conclusive of what?" I asked.

"His symptoms aren't due to a cervical disc problem. There are no obvious cord lesions to explain them. He has wasted muscles in his shoulders, arms, and legs, and twitching muscles on his face."

"You've done a partial EMG and two physical examinations, and now you've seen the other reports," I said. "What's wrong with him then?"

"In my opinion, he has a motor neuron disease— ALS. Many people call it Lou Gehrig's disease. There's no definitive test for it, so you eliminate every other diagnosis first. Since I don't know Mr. Thomas, I don't know how he'll react when I tell him. I need your help in telling him."

I held my breath before I spoke because I could hear my own heart thudding in my ears. Even though I suspected early on that George had Lou Gehrig's disease, it was devastating to hear from a doctor. My heart ached for us as I saw visions of the struggles ahead. I had once nursed Lou Gehrig's patients. The memories of the stale urine and dirty diapers of those old men with empty, withered faces and bodies, and their inability to help themselves, made me cringe. *Oh, no, not my Gentleman George!* I wasn't sure I was up to the awful challenges that lay ahead. As the hair on my arms bristled, I felt only terror.

"Tell him what you think is wrong, and ask him how much he wants to know. Give it to him straight. Considering the potential outcome, you might ask him if he wants a second opinion."

When George didn't appear, I asked if I could go to the examining room and help him dress.

"Of course," he said. "I didn't realize he needed help. He's in the third room on the left."

When I knocked on the door and opened it, George was sitting on the examining table, one foot on the floor, the other dangling from the table, as he tried to button his shirt. He'd been struggling so long, his hands shook, and his fingers were twisted and contorted. He was a meticulous dresser. Even his military records made note of it: "His appearance is always neat as a soldier." He would never go out with his shirt unbuttoned.

I closed the door and hugged him tight. As the

tears filled my eyes, I continued to hold him until I could control myself. "George, please let me help. Dr. Noble wants to talk with you."

"Thank you, Phyl. I'm wiped out," he said, his voice weak. He trembled as I buttoned his shirt, damp with perspiration and plastered on his chest. I saw the slow crumble begin. His eyes were moist and dispirited. In the more than thirty years I had known George, I had never seen him cry.

"George, this is what this marriage stuff is all about, helping your buddy until the end. You'd do the same for me." Then I added, "You always joke around and say you're going to push me in my wheelchair one of these days because of my arthritis."

"Yes, but I'm a man." His lower lip turned up in a grin at the corner. "That's my job."

"Oh, stop that chauvinist crap," I answered. We hugged and laughed.

When we returned to Dr. Noble's office, I sat close to George, although he didn't seem to notice my frequent squeeze of his wet hand. His face was motionless, and he sat soldier-like in his chair, as though waiting for inspection by his commander at the parade ground.

"Mr. Thomas, I have reviewed all your test results. My conclusion is that you have a motor neuron disease, ALS, commonly referred to as Lou Gehrig's disease. Its slow and insidious onset starts in your limbs, or the breathing muscles. You have limb onset, more in your arms than your legs. Your breathing doesn't seem to be affected." He continued, "It's a fatal disease that destroys the human nervous system."

Dr. Noble's face was chalk white. I glimpsed his knuckles whiten when he gripped his hands on top of his desk. He squirmed in his chair. Unlike when he first met George, he spoke slowly. "Would you like me to refer you for a second opinion?" I felt despair for both of them, as I saw Dr. Noble's head tilt to his chest.

"No. It doesn't matter what you call it," George said. "I know its bad news. So how long do I have, and what will my life be like?" George didn't blink. He reacted to the news with characteristic level-headedness. He remained stiff and upright as he pulled his hand from mine.

"Probably about six months. Do all the fun things you've wanted to do but haven't done while you still can. The only treatment is the drug, Rilutek, which may extend your life a month or two, though it does have side effects such as kidney and liver damage." Dr. Noble added, "Before you start it, I need to do some tests to check your liver enzymes and kidney function. Even with the side effects, you should consider it."

"You tell me I have six months to live, but if I take a drug that involves more tests to find out what damage the medicine is doing like possible liver damage, I may live two more months, with a lousy quality of life. What the hell nonsense is that?" Then George added, "My liver is working just fine, and it will stay that way until I die."

I watched George's face for any signal that he planned to leave the office. His lips were drawn tight in a thin line that I recognized as controlled anger, his pupils were fixed, and his face looked frozen. He had shut down and wasn't going to discuss anything.

"Why not talk this over with your wife and come back to see me in three weeks, after you've thought about it."

George answered, "My wife's a nurse, and she'll get me all the information I need. There's no need for me to return. Thank you."

We left the office, George walking stiffly upright.

When we approached the car, he patted my arm as if to reassure me, and he then said with a smirk, "Well, I know what's going to be on my death certificate. That's more than you can say."

Then and there, he set the tone for the journey we traveled.

THE BEGINNING

"I'm your blind date and I'm going to take you out in my white chariot."

On July 10, 1970, I watched a slim, medium-build man sprint up the long, cobbled stairway to my white brick row house in Northwest, Washington, D.C. His movements, beneath a neatly pressed and tailored suit, were fluid. He would have blended in with most forty-plus white men on the street except for a full head of black hair that made him wickedly handsome. I was attracted to him immediately, mesmerized by his large, sapphire blue eyes.

My blind standard poodle, Princess, raced me to the door, and I leapt over her to avoid falling. I heard a loud whistle. George stared wide-eyed through the glass door, watching this gymnastic act. He probably expected me to land, splay-legged, on my fanny. Fortunately I was wearing a mini-skirt that gave me flexibility. Besides, I had had plenty of practice jumping over Princess.

"Hi," he said when I opened the door. "I'm George

Thomas, your blind date, and I'm going to take you out in my white chariot." When I saw the dingy white Dodge van with a dented fender, I thought, *This guy has a beautiful smile and a playful sense of humor. So far, so good.*

Later that evening, after dinner with friends who had arranged our blind date, we shared our stories while sitting on my back porch under the stars, sipping scotch and water, enjoying the fragrances from the hanging baskets of petunias and the Sweet Elysium hedges bordering the driveway. He already knew I was a divorced mom and a professor at George Washington University. When I added that I grew up in the rough and tumble of Boston foster homes and an orphanage during the Great Depression, he stared at me, open-mouthed. It was a lot for him to take in.

As we talked for hours, George asked for more scotch. We were so comfortable with each other, yet I could feel his loneliness. Just six months earlier, he had returned home from Vietnam, where he'd been a squadron commander for over a year. His wife had found another man in his absence and had moved George to the officers' quarters at Andrews Air Force Base. She'd unilaterally ended the marriage, which also ended his family life with four children.

He told me, "I fought long enough for my country to lose my wife and family." I sucked in my breath to keep from weeping.

Yet he was fiercely proud when he talked about his flying years. As a fighter pilot, test pilot, flying instructor, and veteran of three wars—World War II, the Korean

War, and Vietnam—he earned two Distinguished Flying Crosses, a pilot's most coveted decoration, and eight Air Medals, in addition to many meritorious medals. A man who had accomplished great things, he had suddenly lost everything most important to him.

In 1973, after his divorce was final, George asked me to marry him. His ex-wife planned to move to New Jersey with their children to live with her new partner. I declined his offer because I'd promised myself I wouldn't remarry until my daughter had finished college. When I was younger, I'd struggled, working as a nurse, going to school part-time, and finally completing my Ph.D. by age thirty-five. I was determined to give my daughter better opportunities to build her own future.

George and I remained close, caring friends over the years, but we didn't share a home. In 1987, when my daughter, Phyleen, was preparing to enter medical school with a full scholarship, it was time to think of our future.

From that first date in 1970 to our marriage in 1987, we had waited for our time together. Our plan was for me to continue working full-time until 2003. George had retired from the military and teaching. The year we married, we both sold our homes and bought our ideal place in Great Falls, Virginia—a three-acre haven in the country. It was our time to enjoy an easier life together.

But the next ten years didn't go as planned. My only sister died in August of 1987, three months after our marriage. My birth mother, whom I had found later in life, reacted to her loss by isolating herself in her home in Cape Cod, neglecting herself and her surroundings.

She contacted me and asked for help. For the next seven years, I traveled to Cape Cod from Virginia at least twice a month to check on the support system I'd set up with her neighbor so she could live at home. In 1995, she died.

Later that year, we had a huge shock. Medical tests showed that George had low-grade prostate cancer. In 1996, he chose to have radiation treatment instead of surgery.

A year after he completed his radiation series, I noticed that George hadn't recovered his usual strength and vitality. At times, he seemed less alert. By early 1999, his tennis game wasn't as strong either. He sometimes fell unexpectedly on the tennis court—what he called his 'controlled crashes.' He refused to acknowledge the increasing hand tremors that sometimes caused him to drop his tennis racket while playing.

In August 2000, George finally agreed to go for an evaluation by his internist, Dr. Payne. After extensive testing, Dr. Payne referred him to the neurologist, Dr. Noble, who diagnosed George with ALS.

On Friday, October 13th, 2000, our dreams were smashed.

While we were mindful of Lou Gehrig and his grand baseball career, we had never imagined that Lou would become the third party in our marriage and try to come between George and me.

Like many Americans, George and I enjoyed

sports, in particular, baseball. We'd both lived on the East Coast as teenagers during the 1940s, Boston for me, and New Jersey for George. My team was the Boston Red Sox, and my favorite players were Ted Williams and Dom DiMaggio. George's team was the New York Yankees, who had been strong rivals with the Red Sox for the American League pennant for decades. His favorite players were Lou Gehrig and Joe DiMaggio, famous also for marrying Marilyn Monroe.

In the 1990s, George and I travelled with our tennis friends to Oriole Park at Camden Yard to watch the Baltimore Orioles play the Yankees or Red Sox. I embarrassed George when I stood up and cheered for the Red Sox, waving my old, tattered navy-blue Red Sox cap in the air. Because we were sitting in the Orioles section, I was the only one hollering and cheering. "Hey, lady, sit down," was the cry from the fans around us. George suggested politely that I sit down.

"No," I said. "The Red Sox need all the help they can get."

Of particular interest in these ball games was the Orioles' shortstop Cal Ripken, Jr. who was aiming to break Gehrig's record of 2130 games, the most consecutive games played by a professional baseball player. In September 1995, Ripken broke Gehrig's fifty-six year record by playing in 2131 consecutive games. We were there to cheer with the crowd.

Gehrig's accomplishments on the field as the best base runner in the league and his immense humility made him an authentic American hero. According to Barron

Lerner in his book, *When Illness Goes Public* (2006), *The New York Times* broke a story on the first time ALS was referred to in this way on March 13, 1940: "Remedy Is Found for 'Gehrig Disease.'" The chief neurologist at New York's Mount Sinai Hospital was using an experimental protocol of vitamin E pills and injections to treat patients with ALS. One of his patients was Lou Gehrig, who experienced some improvement in his walking and reduced muscle spasms. Thereafter, in the United States, ALS was and is commonly referred to as Lou Gehrig's disease.

Lou was diagnosed with ALS on his thirty-sixth birthday, June 19, 1939. Two days later Gehrig retired because of his illness. His retirement brought national and international attention to amyotrophic lateral sclerosis (ALS).

On July 4th, 1939, after sixteen years with the Yankees, he was honored at the Lou Gehrig's Appreciation Day which George and his father attended. He gave the following speech for which he is widely known:

> Fans, for the past two weeks you have been reading about a bad break I got. Yet today, I consider myself the luckiest man on the face of the earth. I have been in ballparks for seventeen years and I have never received anything but kindness and encouragement from you fans. . . . So I close by saying that I might have been given a bad break, but I've got an awful lot to live for.

I never met Lou Gehrig, but felt like I knew him intimately. Sometimes I thought about 'Lou and George,' thought about the similarities and differences between them. Their first identifiable change was trouble with their game: Lou with baseball and George with tennis. Lou, known as 'The Iron Horse' for his record-setting consecutive games played, and George, the 'stubborn mule rider,' who rode the mule as a West Point cadet during the football games—claiming he was the jackass on top. Both hid their symptoms from themselves and others. Both shared early symptoms of their legs suddenly buckling.

What happened to this remarkable athlete, Lou Gehrig, to cause his mysterious loss of strength and led him to retire from the game he loved so much? What happened to my husband, George Thomas, a professional military man and highly decorated fighter pilot in three wars? As trained athletes, both paid special attention to their bodies, but they were losing strength in their limbs, falling and tripping for no credible or obvious reasons. Each lost his easy sense of movement. Both protected themselves against the perception of their own vulnerabilities by walling off their symptoms and temporarily going on with their lives.

After playing tennis for forty years, when George lost his arm strength, he pushed harder and took more lessons because he could no longer toss the ball to serve. Similarly, Lou forced himself to train harder, but his performance did not improve and his 1939 statistics were the lowest of his career. His reputation as a fearsome base runner was diminished when he lost control of his leg muscles.

Both were shy, soft-spoken men with great humility, close to their immigrant parents, with high standards and expectations for themselves. Lou helped his mother by doing tasks around the house. When George's father watched George fall off his horse while playing polo for the New Jersey National Guard, he told him, "Son, we won't tell your mother. I'll increase the insurance." More than any person in the world, George revered his father, the first Gentleman George.

Neither Lou nor George would talk about what was happening until they found it in their best interest to drop their facade and gain the knowledge that would help them. What they learned about ALS was frightening and discouraging.

ALS, a rare, fatal degenerative neurological disease, affects the function of nerves and voluntary muscles—those controlled by will and that have power over the limbs and breathing. The disease was first discovered in 1874 by a French neurologist, Jean-Martin Charcot. After doing autopsies on his patients, he found hardening of parts of the spinal cord. He named the condition, amyotrophic lateral sclerosis from the Greek language: "a" for without, "myo" for muscle, "trophic" for nourishment, "lateral" for the location of the dying nerve cells in the lateral spinal cord, and "sclerosis" for the hardening or scarring of these dead cells.

The muscles lose their nourishment and become smaller and weaker. The diseased part of the spinal cord develops hardened or scarred tissue in place of healthy nerves.

Of the two onset types, bulbar (breathing) and limb onset, both Lou and George experienced limb onset, in particular in their legs.

ALS is a difficult disease to diagnose. It is diagnosed through a clinical examination and series of diagnostic tests, often ruling out other diseases that mimic ALS.

After patients are diagnosed, they most often ask: when did this start and how much longer will I live? Unfortunately, because of insufficient scientific research, no one knows the answers to these questions. ALSA, the American ALS Association, reported in 2006 that more research advances into ALS have occurred in the last decade than all the time since Charcot identified the disease. It is still known as Charcot's disease in France, and Motor Neurone Disease (MND) in Britain and Europe.

ALS can strike anyone, but mostly people between forty and seventy. Lou was diagnosed at age thirty-six, George at seventy-six. In 2006, the Institute of Medicine (IOM) reported a relationship between military service and later development of ALS, especially among fighter pilots—George's career.

Approximately 5,600 new ALS cases are diagnosed every year in the United States (fifteen each day), culminating in at least 30,000 at any given time. Also, every ninety minutes an American dies of ALS. According to the ALS Association, Lou Gehrig's disease affects one in 50,000 people. Yet, among some groups of athletes, particularly in contact sports, the rate appears to be higher. As far as is known, it is not contagious. Less than ten percent of cases occur more than once in a family lineage.

Finally, no two people have the same pattern of symptoms and progression, thus making it difficult to find effective treatment approaches. However, almost all patients share the wicked burden of uncertainty, not knowing when their legs will buckle, or when they will choke on their food, not knowing what is going to happen the next day or week or month.

We wanted to get rid of this unwelcome intruder in our marriage, but not if that meant losing George.

We started over again in our lives together—we chose to live well in the face of death.

OUT OF THE ASHES

"This disease will have to take everything from me—but I'm not giving it anything! I will fight it until I can't."

On Friday, the 13th of October, 2000, the autumn colors on the tree-lined parkway blurred as I drove George away from Dr. Noble's office in Fairfax, Virginia. My head hurt as I tried to imagine what was going to happen to George and our life together. George was silent. But the doctor's words raced through my mind in a voice I couldn't quiet. "You have amyotrophic lateral sclerosis," he'd said. "You probably have six months to live. Come see me in three weeks."

I wondered why he'd think we'd want to come back after hearing this news.

When we were almost home, George said, "Phyllis, no more tests or doctors' visits on Friday the 13th." He winked at me, but I was too shattered and weak to say anything.

I drove the car to the front door entrance, stopped for George to get out, and watched him walk up the slate path to the front door. His legs wobbled as he dragged his feet.

"The house is unlocked," I reminded him. "Be careful of the dogs." Augustus the Great and Nicholas the Ridiculous were always eager to greet us and didn't understand that being welcomed by two 120-pound Bernese mountain dogs could hurt. Nicky had blundered into George two years ago and bruised George's left knee joint, requiring a month of physical therapy.

George pushed the heavy wooden door open, and started into the house. I expected him to tell the dogs firmly to "Stop" and "Sit," and they would do just that. They knew George's voice meant obedience, whereas they knew my voice meant hugs and kisses. But without George's admonishment, the dogs nearly knocked him over while they headed for my car.

I opened the backseat car door, and they leapt in for some rough and tumble smooching. I needed their affection to restore my balance. Bred as rescue dogs in the Swiss Alps, Gus and Nicky were handsome, with long, shaggy black hair, white chests, and huge black, white, and tan heads. They loved to nuzzle and to launch themselves on us when we played with them on the floor. Their favorite game was to tackle George when he chased me around the house.

I drove into the garage and began to sob and shake while the dogs barked and jumped. Their agitations jolted me alert. I knew what was going to happen to George––and to us––and I knew he wouldn't be willing to talk about this for a while. I was reminded of John Steinbeck's thought in *Travels with Charley*: "A sad soul can kill quicker than a germ." I vowed that I would smile all I possibly could during this journey neither of us had chosen. George would be devastated if he saw me cry, even though he'd seen me cry many times in the past. He needed me to be strong now.

I played with Gus and Nicky for a few minutes, and then put them in the back corral to run and play with the visiting deer. When I went in the house, I looked for George to see if he wanted company. He hadn't turned on the stereo in the den, which he always did, so I figured he must have gone upstairs to his office. He loved sitting at the antique oak desk I had refinished for him, surrounded by shelves overflowing with books, old *Wall Street Journals*, his computer and printer handy.

I decided to prepare a dinner of French rolls, spinach soup, and a crab casserole. The barking dogs reminded me that it was past their suppertime. I let them in, fed them and scooted them back outside before going upstairs to find George. He was staring out his window at the hills rolling down to the lake where a large clump of brushes provided shelter for the wild animals. The lights from neighboring homes were only specks in the distance. I offered to bring a hot toddy up to him, but he wanted to come downstairs.

As we waited for the food to cook, he said some music would be nice. "Let me show you how to work the stereo, Phyllis. You'll have to do it by yourself soon."

Ouch. He had never let me touch his stereo, his bar, or his computer. Was he checking out already? Goose bumps prickled up and down my arms.

"Sure, George. Just let me finish making your hot toddy and pouring myself a glass of wine."

After dinner I broached the subject of letting other people know.

"I don't know who to tell, or how to tell them," George said, "or if I should tell anyone. I don't think I can play tennis much longer. It's not fair to my partners, so I guess I'll have to tell the guys something. Would you be willing to play for me until I see what my arms are going to do?"

"Of course. But have you looked at the guys lately? Two have had hip replacements, one a knee replacement, and one faints easily when driving. They're just out to have fun, not practice for Wimbledon. Why not continue for a week or two and see what happens?"

I let the dogs back in. They raced to George and licked his face, but he seemed unaware of them. Gus pushed his head under George's hand to get a pet. Nicky squeezed between George's legs from the other side and sat on his feet.

"George, you could look at the list of friends I use for party invitations and decide who and how much you want to share. As a starter, you might make a short list from our tennis roster to tell right away."

He copied some names on a pad of paper. I thought we were making progress until he put his pen down. "You're the talkative one, Phyl. I think you should do the calling."

I didn't cry because I wouldn't have been able to

stop. Once a distinguished military officer and university professor, he lacked the confidence to talk to his friends on the phone. "First, I don't have ALS," I said, "and second, they'll want to tell you, not me, that they'll support and help you when you need them." My chest ached as I watched him.

He slumped in his chair. "Do I tell them I have ALS, and what it is?"

"George, you have blue eyes, gray hair and ALS. Come out of the closet and tell it straight."

He handed me the pad of paper with a short list of his tennis friends.

"I notice your children aren't on here."

"It's been just two months since their mother's death," he said. "I don't want to make their Christmas any worse. We can phone them after the holidays."

"Sure. Perhaps we can drive to New Jersey and spend a day with them." We visited with them infrequently. I hoped no one else would tell them before we could.

The next morning, I wrote a draft script for George to review, and we agreed to talk about it when I returned from work. Then I highlighted all his buddies' telephone numbers in the tennis roster so he wouldn't have to search for them. He decided he would tell only his tennis friends this week. He'd ask them not to share this information, because he'd tell the others later.

When I came home he asked, "Would you listen to me practice?"

"Of course."

I'd never seen George so nervous about talking

to anyone, not even when he had defended his doctoral dissertation. I wondered if I should make the calls and spare him this discomfort. *No,* I told myself. It's important that he do it himself. Important for him, and important for his friends. As he read the script, he was like a kid speaking for the first time in front of his third grade class.

This disease had taken all the starch out of him— all his cockiness and flyboy swagger. I accepted that. His life and his death were up for grabs. As his wife, I would assure him that I would do what he wanted, and that he was free to change his mind as we moved along on this journey together.

The next day, I eavesdropped outside his office as he made his first call. He read his prepared speech slowly, and then I heard a big wallop of laughter from him. I learned later that Craig, his dear tennis friend and West Point classmate had said to him "Well, George, that's okay. We thought you had AIDS." Hearing that, George relaxed. "I guess you're right," he said, laughing again. "It's a blessing I don't have AIDS."

George continued to laugh, and they had an easy-flowing conversation. In addition, he proposed that I would play tennis for him, and he would come down to the courts to watch.

After that conversation, George was able to call the rest of his friends quite easily. In fact, I heard him telling them that he didn't have AIDS, and wasn't that a blessing. He joked with them saying, "Phyllis wouldn't be happy if I had AIDS."

Of course, I didn't say to him that they have

treatment today for AIDS. They don't have any for ALS.

    An eerie silence lived in our home for nearly a week: no music, no television, and little conversation. Instinctively, the dogs didn't bark: they sat close to George and nuzzled him gently. He walked through the motions and rhythms of daily living—eating, reading *The Wall Street Journal*, working on his investments on the computer, and sleeping. He asked me to cancel our scheduled social activities for a week, except for one last tennis game with his buddies, and a dinner the following Friday.

    I kept busy teaching, writing a textbook, running the house, caring for the dogs, and playing tennis with my own friends—and his. I gave him the space he needed to be comfortable while he sorted out his thoughts. However, I felt excluded. I cried into Gus's wooly head late into the night. He was such a gentleman dog. He asked for little in return.

    The silence broke on Friday night, when we returned home from a late dinner with friends. George was wiped out from pushing himself to be engaging and charming with friends who didn't know about his diagnosis. His skin was dry and drawn, his face ashen, and his eyes dull, sinking deep into his eye sockets. As he headed upstairs to get ready for bed, feet dragging, he clung to the wide stair railing with a determined grip.

    After the dogs enjoyed their enthusiastic greeting of rolling on the floor, getting their bellies rubbed, smooching, and hollering, I put them in the yard. While they were chasing around barking at the wind, I dragged myself to my office to listen to phone messages.

The first message was from Joe, another West Point classmate. George hadn't told him the news yet. As I heard Joe's voice, I fell into my chair with a thud. He said that George's sister had called him asking for information on George's pending death. She had told Joe that she was going to call George's children and tell them their father had six months to live. Joe said he tried to talk her out of it, but she had made up her mind.

Throughout the thirty years I'd known George, he'd complained about his sister's attempts to manage his life. It had reached the point where he didn't speak to her after their mother died.

The other phone messages were from two of his three daughters in New Jersey, who spoke too fast to understand. One was barely able to catch her breath because she was weeping. I cried listening to them. In their minds, they were facing the loss of both parents too close together.

I left my office and went to our bedroom where I found George asleep. He looked lifeless and for a moment I was scared. I held my hand close to his face to feel air from his nose or mouth. What I saw of his face was chalk white. He had sunk so deep into the coverlets I couldn't see his chest moving. He had pulled on his dark blue ski cap, something he'd begun doing in early September.

With the first rays of morning light, I knew I had to stay home with George when he got the news about what his sister had done. So I rescheduled my plans for the day.

About 10:00 a.m., I heard George in the shower. It would be awhile before he made it down to breakfast, so I fixed his favorite breakfast of old fashioned oatmeal, orange juice, wheat toast, and strong black coffee. First I would feed him. Then I would address the problem of the phone messages. I knew better than to talk with George about anything until after he'd eaten his breakfast. When he was flying, the crew knew to feed him first, because he was a mean son-of-a-bitch until after he'd eaten.

When he came down around 10:30, tastefully dressed in grey slacks, a long-sleeved cotton shirt, and black loafers, he smelled like Ivory soap, his favorite. With color in his face and a big smile, he looked like Gentleman George again.

The dogs wanted to play and pushed him hard against the wall. Nicky accidentally nipped him on the hand. George reached down, talked to Nicky, and rubbed him on the head. Gus pushed in and got a good pet on the head as he barked for the first time in a week. When George got free, he turned on his music and cranked up the volume. The house was alive again.

Then he saw me. "What are you doing here?" he asked.

"I live here," I said.

"I thought you'd be playing tennis. I hope you don't think I sleep this late every morning." He grinned. "Is something happening that I forgot?"

"No. I thought we could spend some time together

since you've been unusually somber all week."

"Okay, how about later today?"

After breakfast, George worked in his office on his investment portfolio, read *The Wall Street Journal* and *Barron's*, and completed his usual business routines until early afternoon.

I prepared a light lunch with a glass of white wine for each of us, and we ate outside on the deck above the pool, with the dogs tucked in close by. George commented on the leaves slowly losing their brilliance on the maple and ash trees along our horse fences. In the fields rolling down to our lake, the hard-leaved goldenrod flowers, shading from deep golden yellow to almost white, swayed lightly in the breeze. We relaxed as the late October sun shone on the lake.

Reluctant to change the idyllic mood, I encouraged George to enjoy another glass of wine and talk with me. As I expected, we discussed his favorite topic, the stock market, along with his thoughts on some new investments he'd just finished studying. We enjoyed challenging each other and sharing our business acumen, but we invested separately. He was the businessman; I was the sociologist.

Finally, I knew I couldn't put if off any longer, so I asked him to come into my office and listen to a couple of telephone messages from the previous night. I gave him a chair near the machine on my desk, and told him the first message was from his classmate, Joe. Then I turned on the answering machine.

George shouted, "What's he talking about? She's going to do what? Tell my children I'm dying? How did either of them know I have Lou Gehrig's disease? I only told a few special tennis friends!"

As his face turned beet red, he began to shake violently and stutter, which I'd never heard him do before. He hit the machine with such force I thought he'd break it. When he picked it up and prepared to throw it across the room, I grabbed the machine away from him and pushed him into his chair.

I'd never seen George like this before, nor had he ever thrown anything when he was angry. His face looked like a flashing neon light, alternately purple and white. His blood pressure had been elevated recently, and the doctor had asked me to check it at home several times a week. I knew it was up now.

His face was wet with tears when he said, "Whose life is it, anyway? This is my life and death, not hers. By calling my children, she's playing God. She's saying that my children have more claims on me than I have on myself. That's wrong. None of them have any claim on me." He added, "She's so cruel to call my children when they're dealing with their mother's death. This must be terrible for them." His chest was heaving up and down in a frantic way.

To my surprise, he blurted out, "The next thing she'll do is try to move in with us." We both burst out laughing at such a preposterous thought.

While he was joking, I borrowed a quip from his favorite author, Mark Twain: "It is a mistake that there is no bath that will cure people's manners. But drowning would help."

He chortled and said, "I think a gas pipe would be better." I gave him a big hug and told him I was off to the kitchen to get us both some cold water.

When I got back, George was writing a letter to his sister. His hands were flying all over the keyboard. I thought, *This should be a winner.*

When he finished, he came to my office and asked me to read it. He was such a gentleman, I'd never heard him use profanity or deride other people. But his fury showed through in this letter.

"Wow, this letter is hot," I said. "Let it sit awhile, and look at it later. How about listening to your children's messages?"

"I'm too upset to think about that right now. Will you call them and tell them I'm not dying, and explain why I wanted to tell them after Christmas? I can't talk with anyone now. Also, please call Joe and tell him thank you."

"George, I'm not the person to call your children. I already called Joe and expressed your thanks. He was uncomfortable being caught between you and your sister, since they've been good friends for some time."

George said, "He probably knows more than he's saying. I expect he's part of the grapevine that operates so quickly. I'll call the girls."

He listened to the messages from his daughters and called them to reassure them he wasn't dying and that he'd planned to call them after the holidays because he didn't want to add to their burden. I heard the sadness in his voice when he tried to help them understand his decision. They were not consoled.

Eventually, he picked up the angry letter and rewrote it more in line with the real Gentleman George. He finished it by saying that he and I planned to enjoy the last few years of our lives together and that he wished that she not interfere or influence our lives in any manner. He said he did not want her to try and contact him at any time.

After I read the letter, I said to George, "I'm sorry for the pain this has caused you. I'm glad you're able to let this go now."

"I like my life the way it is and the way I live it," he said. "I don't want a relationship with her. I made my peace with all of this, years ago."

What mattered most was that George showed signs of rejuvenation when he said to me before going upstairs for a nap, "This disease will have to take everything from me—but I'm not giving it anything! I will fight it until I can't."

Like the phoenix, the mythological bird that ascended from the ashes of its own destruction, George took flight again.

LOOKING FORWARD

"No resuscitation, no CPR, no ventilator. When I'm ready, just let me die peacefully at home. Promise me that."

Standing at the kitchen sink, drenched in sweat from crying, I watched the blue heron preening herself as she sat on top of her high white perch, close to the edge of the lake. A gaggle of Canadian geese were honking and chasing around as they dug in the grass for food.

I loved all our familiar creatures: the deer who visited the dogs and fed from the special garden I planted for them so they wouldn't eat my azaleas; the variety of birds I fed with the many bird houses spread throughout the fields; and our favorite woodpeckers who tried to move into our attic every mating season by poking holes in the side of our cedar house.

I wondered how I could make George comfortable during his remaining six months. I tried to imagine how we would manage so that he would be as peaceful as possible. But the thought of leaving our home overwhelmed me. I didn't know if I could manage it.

George, who had gone to sleep in exhaustion after talking with his children, woke up from his nap only after the sun had set.

While I was preparing dinner, George came into the kitchen, sat on a bar stool at the kitchen island and said, "I'd like a Bushmills and water with no ice." His face lit up with a huge grin as I jerked my head around in his direction.

I studied his face to get some idea of what he was up to, and asked, "Do you want to go to the Old Brogue Pub, or fix it downstairs?"

He got up and headed downstairs. "Let's go downstairs and have a drink and talk."

George didn't share his feelings and didn't like it when I asked him questions, so I had no idea what he was planning. He would tease me and say, "Living with you, Phyllis, is like being in a continuous interview."

George managed his bar, his pride and joy, because he designed it to be similar to his father's bar. When we moved in, he replaced the existing bar with a six by three-foot top of antique oak, a double sink, matching glass racks above, and a mirror on the long wall behind. When friends visited, they enjoyed discussing with him all his bar tending treasures, which he had picked up in his many travels while in the Air Force, and the wide range of whiskeys and liquors. But he wouldn't keep wine in a man's bar. Knowing how fussy he was, I didn't even clean it.

I prepared a plate of cheese, grapes, crackers, and wine for me, and put the dinner I was preparing in the refrigerator. Something felt weird, but I decided to go along with him. When I made it downstairs, he was sipping a Bushmills Irish Whiskey, sitting in his favorite black leather chair with his feet up on the brick platform in front of the wood-burning, black potbellied stove. Smelling the heavy earthy scent of the burning wood and seeing the dogs cuddled close to his chair pushing to get head rubs helped me relax. For a few moments I forgot what had happened during the last few days.

I put the tray of food down on the platform and gave him the wine to open. While he opened it, he asked, "Do you think I am going to die in six months?"

Hello? What is going on? Is he serious?

"No, I don't, " I answered. "Do you?"

"No. I know I have a fatal disease, but I still feel healthy enough to live for quite a while. How does the doctor know how long I will live?"

"He doesn't." I said. "That's his best guess based on his experience working with ALS patients and reading the available statistics from people who have already died." I added, "Would it be helpful to you if I put together information about ALS so you could get an idea of what to expect?"

I took the glass of wine he offered me, which was full to the brim. *Wow,* I thought, as I grabbed some food.

"Yes. Thanks, Phyl. I'm not ready to die. Six months is no time at all. We have so much to do in that time. First, we have to move. I don't want you alone in this big house after I'm gone. There'd be no one to take care of you."

Pleased that George was sharing his thoughts,

I asked him where he wanted to go. "I think we should move back to McLean and find a one-level rambler," he said. "I won't be able to do the stairs here much longer, and there isn't any way we could remodel this house. We need to start looking soon, and get this house ready for sale."

I felt like the bottom of my stomach had exited. I excused myself and headed to the bathroom before I vomited. This was not what I wanted to hear. Give up our special home of fifteen years, our labor of love? But I knew we faced a tough struggle, and I had to make this as easy as possible for him. Still, I didn't understand how selling one house, buying another, and moving were the best strategy for anyone with a six-months death sentence. I knew I couldn't do it all myself.

I sat on the toilet and sobbed. Fighting to control myself while I counted to fifty, I breathed slowly and deeply. My heart began to slow and I felt my shoulders un-hunch. I returned to find George on his second Bushmills, relaxed and enjoying the dogs.

"You want more wine?" he asked.

"No, thanks. I'm still enjoying this one."

He quickly jumped into his argument again. "There's another reason we have to move soon. I want to die at home." He added, "I don't want people standing around my bed watching me die in a hospital. I want a stress-free death and for only you to be there. Promise me that."

Phew. I felt like a boulder had hit me. What was going on?

"Let's talk about this later," I said. "But I promise you a comfortable death at home." I teased him and added, "But if I go first, you have to promise me that I'll die at home."

George laughed. "Well, I don't know if I can make you that promise. I'll have to think about it."

"I'm teaching all day tomorrow, so would you go online and see what houses are available in McLean?" I asked. "Since you plan to be around for awhile, you may want to look for a townhouse with an elevator. That would be comfortable for you and easier for me."

He returned quickly to the issues bothering him. "I need you to promise me that I'll have a peaceful death with no suffocating, choking, or any form of violent death," he continued. "I saw enough violent death in war, and I want a peaceful death. I want to be conscious when I die."

Wow! Did he think I was a god who controlled all life and death events?

He must have been reading my thoughts. "You're a nurse and you can manage this," George said.

"After you read the material I put together, let's discuss this in more detail. Is that all right for now?" I asked. "I promise you'll be comfortable and die at home."

"I trust you, Phyllis, to do what I've asked."

"You can trust me, George," I replied. "Perhaps you want to think of who you want as a back-up person, if, for some reason, I'm not available."

I felt overwhelmed by the responsibility he was giving me—to love him, protect him, and care for him while he lived and died with this devastating, cruel disease.

My stomach danced again. "I'm going upstairs to fix dinner," I said. "Would you like me to put on the financial news?" I wanted him to eat before having more Bushmills.

"Thanks, that would be great."

By then I knew he was burned out from all the emotional events of the day. For him to share his feelings and fears about his death took two Bushmills, his usual was one in the evening.

A week later I gave George a notebook with specific information to read before he made his final decisions. In a teasing voice, he said, "My God, woman. Do I have to read all this? I thought they didn't know anything about this disease."

I told him to prepare for a pop quiz the following week.

"When you're reading, look at the material on the local ALS chapter," I said. "They're having their first fundraising walk in two weeks in the District. Maybe we could attend. It sounds like an active chapter."

"No, thanks. Why don't you go," he said. "You're good at that stuff."

"I think I will. They probably have helpful information and maybe even support groups we might be interested in."

"Not for me," he replied.

After he read all the material, he came to my office a few days later and asked if we could talk. "Sure, let's go downstairs by the fire and be comfortable. I'll bring you a

Bushmills. I just have to finish this letter and send it off."

George didn't react emotionally the way some of us do, including me. He always acted logically. His engineering approach was to think out the problem and find a solution.

By the time I arrived, he was sipping a Bushmills he had prepared. He was busy laying out pages on the table by the side of the hearth. He had underlined in red several paragraphs with his strategies and decisions that he wanted to share.

"I've written down my instructions on all the important issues. I think we need a lawyer to put these in some order that will protect the both of us so that no one can interfere with what we want."

"Did you decide on a back-up person to me, if needed?" I asked.

"Yes. I'll call Phyleen and ask if she will help, if needed." George continued, "I have written a statement that my sister and children are prohibited from any consideration of my life or death."

"Do you plan to share that information with them? Even though you don't see them very often, they may expect to be informed." I added, "Whatever you decide, it is important at some point that you let your family know."

"Why? I don't know them well enough anymore, nor do I trust them enough to share this with them." He added, "You and Phyleen are my family. You have my power of attorney in everything. I expect our lawyer will explain all the necessary documents."

"I'll call her tomorrow for an appointment. Perhaps you can outline your specific decisions and any questions to ask her. The more specifics you can give her, the easier and faster she can put together a document that reflects in detail what you want." I continued, "I don't see on these papers if you want extraordinary means to be used to resuscitate you if you stop breathing."

"No resuscitation, no CPR, no ventilator. When I'm ready, just let me die peacefully at home. Promise me that."

"While you're planning our course for the next few months, I need to say that I can't get this house prepared for sale, find another place, and move in six months. I'm still teaching full time and the holidays are fast approaching. I think we'll probably have time to sell and move by midsummer. But first, we have to find another place."

"Well, maybe. But we need to move as soon as possible."

"No, we don't. We can move downstairs. We have a full bath, bedroom, kitchen, bar, living room, and the doors open directly to the pool. You can walk around the yard to get into the car without climbing any stairs."

"I'm sorry to push you, but I don't want you here alone when I'm gone," George repeated.

I jumped up and hugged him, feeling heat from his body that suggested exhaustion and defeat. I cried into his shoulder feeling like I had let him down by not understanding how important it was to him that I be safe. For George, his biggest concern was how to ensure I would be protected and safe after he was gone. I made a note to call our realtor in the morning.

The following week we met with our lawyer and finalized the documents to create a marital trust that would protect our assets, as well as provide him assurance that he would enjoy the quality of life that he wanted, that he would die a peaceful death at home, and that I would be protected from any challenges from his family.

It was important to me that he knew he was in charge of all the decisions affecting him, and that he was free to change his mind at any time.

George had taken many hits in his life, but no matter the hit, he always managed to take control of his life.

THE MAGIC CONTINUES

"The magic continues. And thank you for all the wonderful years.
Happy Anniversary, Love, George"

After looking by myself at seven one-level rambler homes in McLean for two weeks after work, I decided we wouldn't be moving soon. Every home would require major renovation of bathrooms, bedroom, kitchen, and the addition of at least one ramp to accommodate a wheelchair. Compared to our contemporary open house with twelve-foot ceilings, the older rambler houses had eight-foot ceilings, plus small windows that made the houses seem dark and claustrophobic. The smell of mildew, moldy carpets caught my attention, as these could possibly be harmful to George's lungs. PALS (People with ALS) were subject to respiratory issues, as the disease progressed.

Teaching full time, I wasn't able to plan and supervise the renovations that would be required. And George couldn't help. Plus, after talking with the realtors, I realized the financial considerations were more than we could afford at the time. Knowing George, if he saw these homes, he would argue that we would have to raise the eight-foot ceilings before we moved in. One reason he liked our home in Great Falls was its openness and cheerful, airy spaces.

He would joke and say, "We live in a glass house, but it sure costs a lot to heat." We had ceramic, wood-burning stoves on two floors to boost the heat from the two electric heat pumps.

But as luck would have it, in November a friend told me about a new townhouse development under construction in McLean that included an option to add a private elevator. After riding the elevator in one of the finished four-story townhouses, I gave George all the material to read, and invited him to go with me to see one. To my surprise, when he rode the elevator, he decided immediately that we should move there.

"Even if I die before it's finished, you will be safe and comfortable here after I'm gone," he said.

My belly hurt when he said that. Damn. Why couldn't I get where he was instead of being stuck struggling with giving up our home and our past life? His major worry was for me. He was much more far-sighted, knowing how important it was for us to take care of each other. Our decision to move had to take into account both of our lives—now for him, and later for me.

In two days we'd put a deposit on one of the townhouses that would include a private elevator. However, it wouldn't be completed until August 2001—ten months away.

We moved downstairs in our home, and postponed selling our home until after the holidays, when I would take a leave of absence from teaching to prepare the house for sale and be company for George in the country.

As the holidays approached, I reminded George of the local ALS chapter's Christmas party. This would be his first chance to meet other people with ALS since he was diagnosed.

After I told him about the extensive resources provided to help ALS families, he reluctantly agreed to go to the party with me. I'd learned that the ALS 'Loan Closet' held wheelchairs, shower chairs, bedside commodes, suction machines, and other equipment donated to the chapter by families of deceased members so that others could use them.

While driving to the hospital for the party, we chatted about our upcoming trip to the mountains in two days to join our daughter and her family. George was anxious to leave before the predicted snowstorm. As a former command pilot, he was uncomfortable with someone else at the wheel, especially me, if the weather was bad.

As we entered the hospital auditorium, decorated with fresh pine wreaths and lights, and Christmas music playing in the background, I saw people signing up at an unattended desk. I asked them if this was the ALS party.

"Yes, welcome. I'm Pat and this is my husband, John," Pat said.

After I introduced us, several other people joined

the line using walkers and canes. George took one look at them and tugged on my sleeve to come with him into the hallway.

"Phyllis, we're at the wrong party," he said. "These people are sick."

"Yes, they are sick, George. And so are you. Remember, this is an ALS party. You all share this wretched disease."

"Am I going to look like them?"

"George, I don't know. If you want to leave, we will. But I think we should meet the people, and listen to their experiences with ALS."

"Promise me I'll never look like this, drooling and asleep in a wheelchair with a bag on my leg. I love life, but that isn't life."

"George, I promise you'll be comfortable and die at home." Our new life began with more promises than I knew how to keep.

I added, "We can sit in the last row and leave at any time. It's up to you."

He agreed to stay and sit in the back. As he grumped at me, I hugged him and put his nametag on his favorite worsted tweed jacket.

George became more comfortable as he watched people greeting others eagerly, hugging each other and enjoying themselves. To my surprise, he began talking to the people who were sitting in their wheelchairs, with their oxygen equipment and urine bags hanging on the side.

Then he walked around the large room and found an exhibit of equipment, including the Hoya Lift, special wheelchairs, and other devices. His engineering curiosity got the better of him. He talked with the rehabilitation therapists, specifically about the electric and hydraulic mechanics of the Hoya Lift.

They showed him how the caregiver operates the manual hydraulic lift that is in the form of a sling made out of heavy material to transfer the patient from a wheelchair to a bed, or any other place. The manual lift required more people, skill and effort than the electric lift that was controlled through an electric hand control.

When I met up with George, I asked how the hydraulic lift worked because it looked familiar to me from my days as a nurse caring for ALS and other bedridden patients. I wanted to get him talking about his adventure walking around the auditorium.

"You don't weigh enough to handle this lift, Phyllis. I don't want you doing that," he said. "I'm going to leave this world before I get tied up in all this stuff."

"Oh, George, don't forget Shakespeare's wisdom. 'Though she is little, she is tough.' I've used this equipment before."

We left the party two hours later after agreeing to attend the next support group meeting for ALS patients and their caregivers in January 2001. It was the start of a special journey for us in finding new friends and support for over two years.

Two weeks later, I drove us to the same hospital

building to attend the January support group meeting. Snow was swirling in every direction, visibility was poor, and George navigated the entire ride. I parked at the auditorium entrance and took him inside to a chair in the foyer to wait while I put the car in the four-story hospital parking lot. When I returned, George was walking around in the corridor peeking into different rooms.

"Did you find the meeting?" I asked.

"Yes, in this room. There sure are a lot of sick people here," he said.

We went inside and were met by the group leader and social worker, Robin, who smiled at us with natural warmth, extending her hand in welcome. The large room had windowed walls, and I could see light snowflakes land and adhere on the windows in star-like designs for a few seconds. I sensed George's jaw tighten when he learned the group leader was a social worker. He had an aversion to them.

I found us a seat where he could see out the windows. I knew he appreciated the natural light because he smiled as he sat down and looked at the snowflakes making a design on the windows. There were twenty-six seats around the long conference table; many of them were already filled with middle-class white males and females, appearing to be in their late fifties and early sixties.

Off to the side there was a smaller table with drinks and snacks. I noticed that several women brought desserts and added them to the others. I smelled hot coffee and asked George if he would like something to eat, or a warm drink.

"No, I have the water you brought. That's enough for now."

I went off to get coffee and an oatmeal-raisin cookie, one of my favorite treats that I hadn't time to make since George became ill.

The meeting started at 2:00 p.m. with Robin thanking us for coming, especially on this stormy afternoon that hadn't been forecast. She encouraged us to get some drinks and snacks to bring to the table. She introduced herself and several of her colleagues from the ALS chapter and asked them to say a quick word about their work. Then she invited all of us to go around and introduce ourselves and to share our story of living with ALS.

At first, uncomfortable talking to strangers about his illness, George told the group when we went around the table to introduce ourselves, "My name is George Thomas. My wife will speak for us. She does all the talking in the family."

The men thought he was hilarious. Some of the women frowned. I tickled him under the arm of this sweater so that he let out a yelp. The group relaxed as everyone, including George, shared their stories and experiences with ALS.

George needed male connections, and since most of the ALS patients were men, sixty and over with military backgrounds, with women helping them, he found common ground.

When the meeting ended, a few men came over to talk with George to welcome him and to hear his story. I sneaked out to get some coffee to leave them alone, hoping he would be more comfortable. It worked.

From the other side of the room, I watched how they joked and teased the way men do, patted each other on the back as they become familiar and comfortable with each other. When we left, he said, "Be sure to put the next meeting on my calendar."

Eventually, George was able to open his heart to new friends in the support group. To one meeting he brought socks that stretched easily, which I had found at Hecht's department store at Tyson's Corner. After much joking about their problems with putting on socks, George formed an email group with some of the men so they could help each other with what the disease demanded— appropriate clothing such as shirts with Velcro closing instead of buttons, sweat pants that stretched and were easy to pull up and down, plus technology and tools that provided relief and comfort. It was also an opportunity for the men to share their illness through reaching out to others like them.

The problem of having someone put on someone else's socks became a point for discussion in our monthly support group. The topic became 'socks du jour.' The men couldn't hold their legs up, or extend them so that we helpers could ease the socks over their feet, and the material wouldn't stretch enough for us to accomplish this cumbersome act for someone else. There were no 'sock tools' or 'sock helpers' anywhere.

At the beginning of some meetings, each of the men put their legs on the meeting table, chorus girl style, to show off their latest socks that were supposed to stretch with little effort. They'd found these on the Internet. Jokes abounded as they shared the burden of feeling alone with this horrible disease.

For the next meeting the men decided—with George as organizer—that they needed to have shoe races to see if there were any special tricks about putting on shoes or special types of shoes to buy. Some women had already found shoes with Velcro closing that made it easier for them to care for their husbands. All the men expressed their concern to find ways to make dressing a more manageable activity for them and their caregivers.

Several months later at another meeting, we had visitors from Leicester, England—an adult son, Simon, who had ALS, or Motor Neurone Disease (MND) as it is called in England, and his father, John. The son had told his father that before he died he would like to visit America. The son's mother and grandmother had died of MND. During their visit, they spoke with everyone individually, as they listened to the members' stories and shared their own.

We all enjoyed their crispy British accents as they told stories about the famous movie star, David Niven, who died from MND. Most people thought Niven was American, but he was British and brought considerable attention to the disease and the need for research. John gave all the PALS a blue and gold pin in the shape of a thumb's up to wear in their lapel. It was a symbol of fraternal brotherhood.

After they returned to England, John wrote an article, "It's the same the whole world over," for an MND publication that he sent back to Robin.

John wrote how he and Robin set up the meeting room beforehand, something he was used to doing in Leicester for his son's meetings, and laid out the food and drinks that Robin had provided. He included with the article a picture of the sixteen PALS with their thumbs up, and their caregivers. He described the act of taking the picture of the group: "Then they got in a close huddle with Simon, my son, in the middle."

He mentioned short segments about several of the PALS: the man from Somalia cared for by his neighbor; the woman who had been in London during the war in the WACS and had visited the House of Commons on June 6, 1944 when Winston Churchill announced 'Operation Overlord'; and Gentleman George, who had a penchant for Bushmills Irish Whiskey. John finished the article this way: "What can you say about these wonderful people? I am humbled by them from both sides of the Atlantic . . . and although I didn't want MND in my life, I have to recognize how it also enriches me."

When Robin shared this publication with us at the next support group meeting, you could hear the lengthy silence as we all read it. We felt that we had been enriched by our friends around us and by these visitors from England.

The support group showed George that he had become part of a community in a way he hadn't experienced before. The victims of ALS all had the same diagnosis. They didn't walk alone. George's life grew richer from this experience as he connected with more people. He reached out constantly to help his fellow travelers. It was a brotherhood that he took as seriously as his West Point classmates.

A few months later at the support group meeting, George shared a story of a dumb thing he did. By mistake, he ordered twelve copies from Amazon of Benjamin Graham's big book, *Security Analysis*, instead of ordering one. His nervous fingers had accidentally hit the numbers one and two so that the order read twelve copies. When the UPS man delivered the books, he had trouble lifting the package from his truck. George was flummoxed. He asked the driver, "What are you doing with that big box? I only ordered one copy."

Amazon wouldn't take the extra copies back, so everyone who visited us for the next week or two went home with a bulky copy of Benjamin Graham's *Security Analysis*.

A few weeks later several of the wives and I decided to attend a newly formed support group for caregivers only. I suggested we meet for lunch at 12:30 the next Sunday and then go to the meeting at 2:00 p.m. close by at the hospital annex. One middle-aged Asian woman was so bereft because she had never heard of this disease and had no family in this country. They had been here two years. Six months after they arrived, her husband was diagnosed with bulbar type ALS that was progressing swiftly. They wanted to return home, but were afraid he wouldn't survive the trip.

Immediately, the group rallied around to hug her and offer to help in any way. Each woman shared her story and by the time we had finished lunch, we felt a bond of sisterhood that we knew would nourish all of us as we travelled this journey together. I realized that my story was far less burdensome than the other stories I heard. Two husbands were close to needing ventilators to assist their breathing; another was scheduled in two weeks to go into the hospital for insertion of a rubber feeding tube in his abdomen. George was still able to walk, although he needed help eating when he was tired. He had no breathing problems.

Everyone's story was different because there were no shared set of symptoms or pattern of progression with this disease, making it difficult to know what to expect and prepare for. The uncertainty was troubling to everyone.

When we arrived at the meeting, five other women were there talking and sharing their experiences. The leader had not arrived. Unfortunately, the tiny meeting room was in the basement with no windows and the air smelled of dead fish. When the leader arrived she was embarrassed because this was the second unsuitable room she had been given. We met for a short time, exchanging email and phone addresses so that we could be in contact until a more appropriate meeting room could be found. I offered a meeting room at the Army Navy Club that we belonged to.

None of us would have traded our husbands or wives in because of what had happened. But we all had dark moments, and the ALS support groups provided a place where we could talk without fear of being judged about how we handled the problems we faced. Caregivers do feel anger, not at the ill person, but at the circumstances that seem stacked against them and their loved one. I was mad at my whole life, and angry because we'd lost the dreams we had for our retirement and life together. Dreams that we'd worked so hard for, now gone. Others shared their sorrows, and agreed it was something we could never be prepared for. We listened to each other with respect and empathy, realizing that listening sometimes helps people as much as anything else.

During the more than two years we attended the support group, many of George's friends died. There were usually fifteen PALS along with their caregivers, at each meeting. George's disease progressed at a slower rate than most, and he was able to walk in and out of the meetings unless it snowed, when I insisted he use the travel wheelchair.

During the course of our meetings, we usually met many of the same people, but deaths happened many times, which upset George. In particular, two of his male friends died in hospitals after they'd made clear to the support group they wanted to die at home. One man, Mike, who lived alone with bulbar ALS, which affects the diaphragm—the flat muscle that expands and contracts the lungs—struggled with breathing problems early on. He brought his computer to the support group as his speech became indistinguishable because it was programmed so that he could speak to the group. He and George quickly developed a fondness for each other and they shared a love of music, especially old time jazz. They exchanged emails, CDs and articles that they thought the other would enjoy.

When he didn't appear at one of the meetings, George asked Robin, our leader, to trace him down. George had tried, but Mike hadn't answered his emails. When we learned at the next meeting that Mike had died in the hospital a few days earlier, George dropped his head to his chest and turned his shoulder so no one could see his face. We were all quiet for about fifteen minutes as the sad news settled in.

On the way home, George leaned into the car window as his face and body shook from the news about his friend, Mike. I turned up the heat because he had recently complained of feeling cold. This, plus the death of his friend, probably made him feel wiped out. There was a hush in the car until we were almost home. There was the sound of waiting. In a meek voice, he said, "Please don't let me die in a hospital, no matter what happens."

"I promise you, George, as long as I'm breathing,

that won't happen. Phyleen has promised the same. I'm very sorry about Mike. He was so passionate about his wish to die at home." I added, "Unfortunately, he lived alone and his daughter didn't live close by. It must have been hard for her to put him in the hospital."

Over time, George became very fond of Robin, our social worker. This was another change in George's acceptance of people's work that he didn't understand. He told many people about 'his' social worker, Robin. He sought out ways to be useful to her by offering to set up a complete email file so we could all contact each other between meetings. He also made sure I prepared drinks and dessert for the meetings, as well as helped to set up the room. He supervised, entertaining us with his humor while we worked together. This was the new George.

The companionship shared by these men encouraged a spirit of empathy. They shared each other's pain. This companionship brought out George's compassion which otherwise wasn't often visible in this silent man. He came out of himself with these people because they all did their very best, as they suffered and were gradually stripped of their independence. Everyone was equal in the room. His life in the military was one of authority, control, rank, and status. With this disease, none of that mattered. Everyone was in charge; no one was in charge.

At the end of April, 2001, we put our house up for sale and prepared to celebrate our wedding anniversary, May 1, by traveling to Nashville, Tennessee. There we would attend a special soccer game in George's honor, planned by Coach Edward, our son-in-law. Our five-year old granddaughter, Claire, was playing.

Before we left, George gave me three CDs and an anniversary card with a couple dancing on the front. The handwriting on the card was decipherable but shaky and showed the struggle it had been for him to write it:

> *Pops Stoppers will cause your feet to tap.*
> *Eine Kleine Nachtmusik will soothe.*
> *Franz Schubert's Unfinished Symphony will remind you that our symphony is not finished yet*
> *. . . .*
> *The magic continues. And thank you for all the wonderful years. Happy Anniversary. Love, George*

I didn't know at the time that this would be the last card George ever wrote to me.

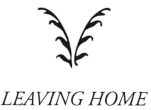

LEAVING HOME

"Now, who's going to look after Phyllis when I'm gone?"

When we returned from Nashville and I saw the ugly *For Sale* sign in our front yard, I nearly lost control of the car. I came close to hitting the white country fence at the entrance to our circular driveway. That scared George, as he grabbed the car door handle. He probably thought I was tired from driving the entire thirteen hours.

"You must be tired. I'm sorry I couldn't help you with the driving." Then he added, "What you need is a long bath, a book, and a glass of wine."

That was George's usual explanation for any of my strange behaviors: I must be tired. I knew his explanation of my response would never change, but I do take a lot of baths.

Although I regained control of the car, chills ran through my body when I saw that *For Sale* sign. It threw me back to leaving the orphanage in 1946 where I had lived for at least five years. I was thirteen, and it was a safe place I called home, after traumatic years in foster homes.

Now I had another safe place that was home, and it was up for sale. I tasted the bile in my throat.

My discipline and training clicked in. Quickly, I forced myself to focus and parked the car. George's face returned to its normal color.

"Sounds like a good idea, George." I said. "I'm tired and I do need a bath. I'll unpack the car in the morning. I have to go out early to get the dogs."

Thinking about the dogs caused me to chuckle about the time three weeks earlier when big Gus gave me the worst case of poison ivy of my life. When he saw me standing in my swimsuit at the pool, he came running through my bare legs after he had been in our large three-acre field chasing geese and rabbits. Poison ivy vines ran rampant throughout the fields and their oil clung to his long, black coat.

I tried using calamine lotion to dry the weeping blisters, and Benadryl to reduce the itch, but I was in misery. I called the dermatologist for a cortisone shot to reduce the swelling and discomfort, and took Gus to the groomers to get a real bath to remove the poison-ivy oil. It took two people working for two hours to clean his one hundred-twenty-pound body. It was two weeks before I could sit down without a rubber cushion. There's nothing friendlier than a wet dog with poison ivy.

How embarrassed I was trying to explain to my dermatologist that my dog gave me poison ivy after he had been running in our fields. He raised his eyebrows like he didn't believe my story. I was most uncomfortable sitting on the cold, metal examining table in his office in my underpants. He gave me a shot in my rump and said little. I wondered if he thought I had been frolicking in the fields bare-assed.

A week later when George and Gus took their usual walk down the country road as part of their exercise program, I realized they had been gone longer than usual. I jumped in my SUV to find them, knowing they travelled the quiet country road where only neighbors drove. When I curved around the bend in the road, about three-hundred feet ahead, I saw George sitting on the ground in the sun. His legs were crossed in his usual meditative pose. Gus looked like a dead cow at his side, his extravagant, black body sprawled out on the grass. He lifted his head off the ground as soon as he heard the car. George barely moved from his meditative pose. My heart filled with sadness at this pathetic sight, but I was relieved they were safe.

I parked my SUV and ran over to him. "What happened?"

"I don't know. Gus lay down and wouldn't get up. I told him you would come soon."

"Are you okay?"

"I'm tired." He added, "I don't think we should do these walks anymore."

"Would you like me to help you up?"

"Please."

I pulled George up from the ground, and struggled to settle him in the car. His legs kept folding when I tried to lift him into the front seat of my SUV. I realized that he had slipped to another plateau. His legs had lost more control. Then I went to work on the dog.

Gus was unable to lift himself off the ground, so I rubbed his hot, white belly—his favorite rub—as he rolled on his back with four white feet in the air. If I could get him relaxed, I could stand him up and lift him into my SUV with a little help from him.

Fortunately, it worked. After I'd helped him stand up and stumble to the rear of the car, we did the old drill: I showed him where to put his front paws. Then I called one, two, three, and grabbed him from the rear, hoisting his hind legs into the SUV as I pushed his body forward. We had done this drill many times as his back legs became weaker.

Then I took my two wounded soldiers home.

Augustus the Great (Gus) was the soul of our household. As a gentleman dog with an immense capacity for wisdom, he knew his family well. Being a great listener, who talked very little, he helped take care of my heart. Although I tried not to cry in front of George, I cried all over Gus and his wooly head. Sometimes his body shook, I sobbed so hard.

During those sieges, he pressed his body harder into mine. I told Gus everything because George wasn't interested in hearing my tales. He was too exhausted coping with his own travails.

Sometimes when Gus had enough of my talk, he reached out and put his huge paw on my leg. That was his signal to me. "Time to slow down, girl," he was saying. "Calm down." I couldn't stay sad or angry when a great big paw gently grazed the side of my face. He had my attention, dragging me out of my sorrow to show me what he needed: a wonderful belly rub. He restored my balance.

One evening as he and Nicky chased me around the pool, he accidentally pushed me into our swimming pool in my favorite green silk pantsuit. The dogs barked and danced around the pool following me while I swam.

Now, two weeks later, Gus was unable to get up off the ground. His body smelled of loose bowels. I looked into those big brown eyes and for the first time I saw the deep pain he'd managed to mask. I broke into a sweat, a rare experience for me. My face went cold and my gut clenched. I knew I had to get him to Dr. Steve. I gave him Ascripton (Aspirin and Maalox) with some ground meat for his pain, so he could rest until I took care of George. I had been giving Gus Ascripton once a day for more than a year to reduce joint stiffness. George took Ascripton daily for muscle pain.

I woke George and brought him downstairs for breakfast. I suggested that he talk to Gus because I didn't think he'd be coming back to the house. George said little but went over to Gus and thanked him for all the happiness he had brought to our house. "Now, who's going to look after Phyllis when I'm gone?" he earnestly asked Gus.

Hearing that was too much for me. My legs went soft. I left the room, called Dr. Steve, and told him I was coming in with Gus.

Driving Gus to the hospital, I felt tortured. I hadn't

noticed Gus failing so quickly. I was too busy caring for George, and working with the builders and designers on the new townhouse every day—selecting floors, windows, tiles.

Also, I was trying to get the house ready to put up for sale. This meant meeting all the realtor demands: take furniture in this room and put it in another room, take all the family photos off the tables, etc. etc. Anyone who has ever sold a house knows how horrible the experience can be when realtors try to redecorate your house. You are left thinking, *How did I ever live in this horrible place with all this furniture and trash?*

I went into the hospital and found Dr. Steve. He told me he would come out and carry Gus into the X-ray room. The doctor was a physical giant, over six feet tall, muscular, and young. His primary practice was with large animals, so he spent a good bit of time caring for farm animals. I had yet to see any cows in his office, but I had seen a few pigs.

After fifteen minutes, Steve came looking for me and found me crying in my car. He told me I needed to come in and look at Gus' X-rays. When I entered the room where Gus was lying on his side on the stainless steel examining table, he heard my voice, lifted his head off the table and tried to get up.

I ran over to the table and put my arms around him, knowing that I was about to hear some bad news. After I had settled him and me, I looked at the films of his spine with Dr. Steve. It was obvious that Gus couldn't live much longer with any quality of life. We studied the films and saw a massive shadow, the cancerous growth that had fractured his lower spine.

I held Gus' heavy head and thanked him for the happiness he had given us. As I talked to him he weakly tried to lick my hand. I wept into his furry black head. His big brown eyes told me I had to let him go—now.

As I held Gus, Dr. Steve administered the final medicine to end his life and his pain. I couldn't drive for at least an hour. I don't remember how I drove the thirty-five miles home. By then, I was running on fumes.

Nicky was distraught when I returned. He ran to the car looking for Gus. He never recovered from the grief of losing his buddy. He wouldn't touch his food, or let anyone pet him. I called Dr. Steve who prescribed medicine for depression, which didn't help. The next year Nicky developed a debilitating neurological condition that was not treatable. I had to make the decision to grant him death.

I knew George was next.

After our house had sold, during the remainder of the summer, I made arrangements for us to move. Our new townhouse was completed. After we moved in, I needed to clean our house before I turned it over to the new owners on September 14, 2001.

At 7:00 a.m. on September 11, 2001 when the movers pulled into the driveway with their van, I questioned them on the size of the van and the number of workers. We were scheduled for an eight-hour move that would finish no later than 5:00 p.m. I was skeptical about this because I knew George would be worn out by then. Anything later than that would be disastrous for him. I considered taking him to a friend's house, but the workers reassured me that they would finish the move on time.

After they had worked for over two hours, I suggested they take a coffee break in the kitchen. We sat drinking coffee and exchanging funny stories about their past jobs and mine as seasoned movers. Jovial and relaxed, I asked them to load George's bed last so they could put it together immediately at the new house.

George was reading his investment news on the computer upstairs when he learned about the plane crashes in New York City and the Pentagon. He came down to the kitchen and told us what had happened. I thought he must have been dreaming. We turned on the television and viewed the horror, terrified as we watched the reporting of a plane striking the Pentagon.

We didn't speak. We could never have imagined this happening in the United States. We, as a country, had no idea of how vulnerable we were. After a long period of silence watching the news, George said, "In the many years I worked there, we all considered the Pentagon to be a fortress."

Finally regaining my focus, I said to the workers, "Would you like to go home and be with your families? We can do this tomorrow."

They thanked me but declined and we went back to work—but at a much slower pace. George was quiet,

continuing to watch the news. He told me later he was
relieved I was safe. Tuesday was my day to play tennis with
my women friends at Army Navy Country Club. I had
cancelled because of our move. Otherwise, I would have
been on Interstate 395 when the plane hit the Pentagon. I
could have been under the wheels of that airplane.

The movers took many more hours than estimated
because we were all worn thin from the horrible events of
the day. They finished after midnight.

We were both quiet as I closed the door to our new
home. The subject of death was high in our minds. As it
turned out, the horrible attacks in New York, Virginia,
and Pennsylvania overshadowed the trauma of leaving our
first home.

The next week I cleaned our home to prepare for
the new owners. When I was done, I sat with my feet in
our black gunite pool, staring at our lake for the last time.
The deer graciously scooted around, munching here and
there. They reminded me of my young grandchildren
when they visited. The kids bounced around, munching
and grazing like cows, and the younger one rode on Gus's
back.

During the fourteen years we'd lived there, we
made friends with all God's creatures. Many deer came to
the wrought-iron fence at our swimming pool and visited
nose-to-nose with our big dogs, all of them making dancing movements like teenagers with their heads bouncing

and feet tapping. I often fed two majestic red foxes, and the many bird feeders throughout the property housed all sorts of birds. The redheaded woodpeckers drilled holes that became tunnels in our cedar siding and made nests in our large attic, filled with extra stuff from both of our previous homes. George fought with the woodpecker parent, who flew directly at him when George took the nests outside to save them. The woodpecker didn't know who he was up against.

I insisted that George not kill the babies. We put the nests in a protected alcove I had built, and the parents found their babies immediately. Then our handyman, Cheever, patched up the holes on the side of the house, ready for the woodpeckers' next mating session, their next attempt to make a home among our old possessions.

When it was time to exchange papers at the settlement on our home in Great Falls, George was too tired to attend. But he'd already met the new owners. The woman was a trainer and owner of thoroughbred horses, and for this reason she wanted the property to be near a large horse farm. She planned to bring her horses down from upstate New York. She and George enjoyed talking horses. George had been a professional polo player before he went to West Point in 1944 and he also played at the Academy. Our daughter, Phyleen, was a trained equestrian who also owned several horses.

The new owner husband, like our son-in-law, was a lawyer. He was also a Harvard graduate like Phyleen. They had both lived in Eliot House as undergraduates, but they hadn't met. Phyleen graduated a year ahead of him.

Thus, because of these pleasant coincidences, leaving our home was somewhat less painful than it might have been. Later, our grandchildren played with their son when all of us met for dinner at the Old Brogue Pub in Great Falls.

Everyone laughed when our four-year-old granddaughter, little Lorna, asked them, "Did you know you're living in my grandmother's house?"

TALKING ABOUT DEATH WITH YOUR DOCTOR

"You can't keep decorum up for very long with no clothes on."

A year later, we returned to see Dr. Noble to talk with him about George's medical directive. He wanted Dr. Noble to agree to his conditions of care when he moved closer to his death. He wanted to die at home peacefully with no artificial interventions such as a feeding tube, breathing devices, and no attempts to resuscitate him when he stopped breathing.

At bedtime recently, George had begun to talk in his sleep about some of his adventures while he served in the Korean War and Vietnam as a fighter pilot in the Air Force. As he grew weaker, those haunting memories surfaced more often. When my co-author, Dianne Kammerer, and I sat at my dining room table reading galley proofs for our forthcoming textbook, we could hear George upstairs shouting out about horrific incidents he'd witnessed during the wars. He stuttered as he described the violence of those wars, seeing young men die in frightened terror—barely able to breathe before medics could get to them.

There were others with body parts blown off who waited for transport to makeshift facilities. The stench of burning flesh, the fear so clear in the faces of the young men were still vivid in George's mind. He'd earned many meritorious medals and two Distinguished Flying Crosses for rescuing many. He'd made me promise him he wouldn't experience a violent death.

As a Buddhist, George wasn't afraid to die. But it was essential to him that he be conscious and sitting up when he died. He believed that the purpose of life was learning, growing and evolving into a more humane person.

George and I arrived at Dr. Noble's office and sat in the same dismal waiting room as the year before. This time it was nearly empty. When he entered to get George, Dr. Noble seemed pleasantly surprised to see him alive, talking and walking. He smiled broadly as he extended his hand to George. "Mr. Thomas, how nice to see you," he said. Then he asked me to wait there while he examined George.

"I'd like my wife to come with me, if that's all right," George said.

"She can come later, after I examine you," Dr. Noble replied.

I didn't like his answer because George wanted me there. I knew he couldn't hear well since he had stopped using his hearing aids because they made buzzing noises in his ears. He refused to go to the audiologist to have them balanced. Also, he couldn't dress himself without help. I wondered if Dr. Noble thought George would be embarrassed for me to see him undressed in front of another person, or if he thought he would be more successful getting George to agree to some form of treatment, or test, if I wasn't present. Did he think George was some wimpy nerd?

Fifteen minutes later, Dr. Noble found me in the waiting room and said, "Your husband wants you to come to my office while I talk with him. Is that all right with you?"

"Of course it is," I answered, and followed him. When we arrived, I asked, "Where's George? He'll need help getting dressed."

"The last room on the right at the end of the hall."

After I helped George finish dressing, we went to Dr. Noble's office. George's wasn't pleased with this visit and wanted to leave. "There's nothing more to say to him, let's go."

"I'm sorry you're upset. But we need him to look at your medical directive." My guess was that Dr. Noble had approached George about doing more tests.

Dr. Noble was sitting at his polished mahogany desk crowded with tall stacks of paper, pictures of family members, and packets of sample drugs. We sat in the same two seats as we had the year before when he was diagnosed.

"Mr. Thomas," Dr. Noble said, "the extent of atrophy in your leg muscles is less than I expected. You seem to be walking without too much difficulty. But your shoulder muscles are severely affected. I notice you can't raise your arms very high."

"That's right. I'm still struggling to feed myself some of the time. I manage by bending my head down and curving my arms." George added, "Phyllis has to do most of my bathing and dressing, but we're still having a good time. You can't keep decorum up for long with no clothes on."

Dr. Noble half-smiled and continued, "You seem to be stabilized—at a plateau. I'd like to measure the muscle response in your arms. I'll only test a few of your nerves. Also, I'd like to measure the muscle strength in your legs. Are you falling at all?"

"Why do you want to do tests on a man who was supposed to be dead six months ago?" George asked. "How gone is gone? I'm not having any more tests. It's pointless and painful. ALS is a fatal illness. Let's see how fatal *you* are today."

The silence was palpable.

George caught his breath and said, "I came to talk about my medical directive." George asked me to give him a copy.

Dr. Noble's head jerked up. He seemed startled at George's answer. He stared at George, paused, and frowned before looking at the copy I put in front of him. His face appeared frozen as he started to pick up the document. After reading part of it, he said, "I'm not comfortable with this. I'm your treating physician. I think you should take the drug, Rilutek, that I recommended a year ago."

"It's pointless to me to take an experimental drug that has potential serious side effects. I'm comfortable the way I'm living. Why do I want to endure more tests to see what damage the drug's doing to decrease my current good quality of life?" Then George added, "Death isn't my enemy, but these tests and that drug are."

As I watched them talk back and forth, I saw that George's anger seemed to be escalating. His voice became louder and stronger, despite the softness in his voice that had crept in since ALS. I remembered a year earlier when we sat in these same seats. I felt a pang of sadness as I remembered when he had first refused Rilutek. George had walked out of Dr. Noble's office and had refused to return until today when I convinced him he needed to share his medical directive with his physician. He needed his physician's consent if he ever decided to enter the hospice program.

Sitting stiffly in his chair, Dr. Noble read more of the five-page medical directive, saying nothing.

George continued, "I have only so much muscle strength left. I don't want to waste it on more tests. My medical directive states I want to die peacefully at home with no ventilator, oxygen, feeding tubes, or any other such stuff. That is my choice."

I was thrilled by the firmness and resolve with which George informed Dr. Noble of how he wanted to die. I reached over and took George's hand. I could also see he was getting stirred up and that wasn't good for him. He was not a talker, but he was wound up now. Upset at myself for suggesting he come and talk with Dr. Noble, I squeezed his hand to get his attention. He pulled his hand away. I wanted to run out of the room and leave these two men to their arguments.

Tears filled my eyes as I tuned out. I thought back to the many years when I worked as a hospital nurse—how difficult it was for us to get doctors to talk with families and patients about death and dying. As nurses, we were most often the only persons present when patients died. We were the ones who called and talked with the families and had to ask the family for autopsy permissions. Physicians continued to perceive death as failure, especially in this day of high-tech medicine when they could delay death indefinitely.

George stood up, soldier-straight, and turned to face the door. At that point, Dr. Noble, squirming in his chair, bowed his head and looked at the document again. George turned and spoke to Dr. Noble. "My wife knows what I want. Don't fight with her. I love her, but I don't fight with her. Also, our daughter is a physician."

"Do you want me to call your daughter?" Dr. Noble asked.

"Thank you. No. She'd probably agree with you that I should take the Rilutek. My wife's my support person. She'll take care of me."

Dr. Noble looked in my direction. That gave me a chance to ask, "As his treating physician, does that mean you'll be willing to refer him to hospice care if he should need it?"

"Are you considering it now?" he asked.

"No. It's not an immediate plan. Since you are

his neurologist, we may need help later because a referral is necessary to get into the program." I added, "Also, would you please write a prescription for me to give to the Department of Motor Vehicles so they will give me a handicapped-parking sticker? We need that now."

Dr. Noble picked up a prescription pad from his desk, wrote the order and handed it to me. He took a deep breath and said he'd meet George's wishes to the degree that he could. He stood up from his desk to escort us out of his office.

George spoke again, "My wife knows how to work with doctors. She'll make sure I get what I want."

We left the office not knowing if Dr. Noble would help, but George knew I'd keep my promises to him.

As we walked to the car, I said to George, "You know that death isn't a doctor's friend. I'm glad you spoke up and took responsibility for your own life and death." Then I said, "I think Dr. Noble will come through if you decide to enter hospice care. I will call him when and if you decide to make that choice."

HAPPY FIRST BIRTHDAY, GEORGE

"Because of all of you, my dear friends, I know I will have a second birthday."

If your time is limited, every celebration is the greatest. We were celebrating because George had lived an entire year after Dr. Noble told him he probably had six months to live. In the course of a lifetime, how many people get to celebrate their first birthday a second time?

On Sunday, October 14, 2001, we drove with our guests to the 1763 Inn for his birthday party. In the past, October was our month to entertain friends for brunch at the Inn. It felt like coming home again as I breathed in the fresh air blowing off the peaks of Virginia's Shenandoah and Blue Ridge Mountains. Log cabins still covered part of the thirty-three acres. Many sections of pasture—separated by black, wooden fences—were still home to horses and cattle.

The bright sun shimmered on the lake at the bottom of the hill below the Inn. I thought of how many times during the last five years we fed three ducks there, the ones supervised by a bossy, aristocratic swan who sat on her ferociously guarded eggs—several tennis balls.

I found our hostess, Uta, and reviewed the sumptuous brunch menu. Already I could smell the sauerbraten, knockwursts, spicy red cabbage, and fresh breads. I was expecting 120 friends and family members coming from as far as Florida and Ohio, who planned to stay in the log cabins. Making sure everything was in place, I checked the bar and the location of the podium and microphone for George's friends who would probably want to share stories to tease him.

The Professors from Shenandoah University arrived, elegant and smart in their tuxedos, carrying their instruments: trombone, clarinet, trumpet, violin, French horn, guitar, double bass, saxophones, and several percussion instruments. They'd played for us before and were skillful at switching instruments to carry us to new heights. We reviewed the general program for break times, for the cake cutting, and the grand finale.

As our friends arrived, the Professors played a medley of World War II-era dance and jazz pieces—especially songs that Dizzie Gillespie, Louis Armstrong, and Duke Ellington made popular. Soon, people were drinking, eating, dancing, milling around, hopping tables, and hugging, as we always did when we got together to celebrate.

Many children were there too, from little ones to teenagers. They ate hot dogs and drank lemonade, then hollered and squealed as they raced around to play hide and seek in the bright sun and cool breeze. Some sang with the music as they danced with each other on the grass; others danced with their parents on the cabana's wooden floor.

As I scanned this crowd of friends who loved to party, I saw George laughing as people hugged him. I found one of the men and asked him to help George with a drink, because he needed someone to hold his glass and straw. They were all eager to get him one and join him.

Soon George was dancing with the ladies who put their arms around his neck as they swayed with the music. He told them, one at a time, "I don't have any control over my arms and hands. It's possible my hands might land on your fanny."

The women laughed and hugged him, "That's okay, George. But you look so well." He smiled when he told me the story later. "People sure don't know what's going on in someone else's body," he said. I agreed and added, "Yes, but you're still a handsome devil."

Watching the dancing, I remembered what we were told about dating when I was a teenager: "You dance with the guy you brought to the party." George was so busy dancing with all the ladies that I had to drag him away from the women for one dance before he cut his first birthday cake. I realized that Lou Gehrig wasn't in the room. There wasn't a single disabled person in the room. George's radiant face was proof of that.

When he prepared to cut his birthday cake and blow out the one candle, he joked with his friends, "When you lose track of your limbs, your hands and arms become appendages that are more like pieces of luggage you have to drag around."

He bent down to look at his cake. "Phyllis and I are going to cut this cake together and pretend it's our wedding cake that we didn't have because we eloped." He added, "We got married seventeen years after I asked her and she refused. When she called me and finally said yes, I had to ask her, 'Now what was the question I asked you so long ago? I forgot.'" The crowd laughed.

"Thanks for sharing my first birthday with Phyllis and me. I can't believe I'm one year old because sometimes I feel 110." George added, "Yet, we don't view our life as tragic. We know we have limited time, but so does everyone. We're enjoying our lives to the fullest with our family and friends."

He looked down at the cake again. "Because of all of you, my dear friends, I know I will have a second birthday." Before he blew out the one candle on his birthday cake, he told everyone the story of Lou Gehrig who thanked his friends at his farewell address in 1939 by saying, "I am the luckiest man."

George told his friends, "Today, I say the same to you: I feel like the luckiest man with all my friends here to help me celebrate. I thank you."

After we all sang "Happy Birthday" to him and "For He's a Jolly Good Fellow," George blew out the single candle.

But he had one more thing to say before we ate cake. His jaw was tight, and you could read true grit on his face when he added, "I want you to remember that this party is just a rehearsal for the *real* party to come. At my *real* party, I don't want anybody to get up and say what a great guy I was, because that might start a fight. You must all drink, eat, and dance well since I'll be paying for it."

After we enjoyed the cake, I signaled the Professors. They raised their horns to the sky, playing "When the Saints Go Marching In" as we paraded out to the grass and pond. We marched from the cabana onto the grounds around the lake. The swan honked right along with us. As we marched, we sang with mixed voices, "Oh, when the saints go marching in, oh, when the saints go marching in, Lord, how I want to be in that number, when the saints go marching in."

On the drive home after the party, George was overwhelmed. He said, "I never knew I had so many friends, and that so many people liked me." He had been so beaten down after his wife found another man while he was in Vietnam that he deeply felt he had few friends. What a wonderful revelation for him to feel that so many friends loved him.

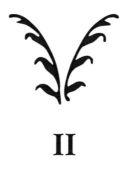

II

NOVEMBER 2001-OCTOBER 2002

TOUGH LOVE

"The next time I fall will be in front of a church, instead of a pub."

In December 2001, we visited George's ophthalmologist for his routine eye exam. Before the visit, his doctor had found a reading table online with a flexible arm attached that would hold George's book and help him turn pages. When he told George about this, I could see the wetness in his eyes as he thanked his doctor. He was excited, and asked me to order the table for him. Fortunately, there were no signs of glaucoma or macular degenerative disease in George's healthy eyes, but he needed an adjustment in his reading prescription.

Two weeks later, I drove George to the optician's office to pick up his new glasses. It had snowed the night before, leaving at least a four-inch blanket of snow everywhere. I bundled up George in his wool ski cap, his old brown leather flying jacket, a bright red scarf a friend knit for him, and winter boots. Only his eyes were visible. He looked as happy as a pig in mud.

Seeing a dusting of snow on the steps to the office, I was concerned there might be ice underneath. There were no other cars around and little sign that people were out shopping. I held George's arm as we climbed up the two medium-sized steps.

George was in a jolly mood, happy to be out doing something real, and getting his glasses. He enjoyed teasing Susan, the optician we had worked with for several years. She told him he looked like an Eskimo. He joked, "I feel like one. It took Phyllis a half hour to dress me, and that's only my snow clothes." He winked at me and tried on his new glasses.

"Come back when you need your glasses adjusted, or just come back and see me anyway," Susan told him as we prepared to leave. "I love your funny stories."

George went ahead of me leaving the office. As I turned to close the outside door, he slipped away from my grasp and fell forward down the two stairs toward the driveway. Luckily he didn't fall into the few cars. My heart stilled. My feet froze. Not again! I ran toward him, saw he wasn't bleeding or having trouble breathing.

He had done his usual trick of rolling up in a ball. He knew how to move with the grace of a snail retreating into its shell. When he'd fallen on the tennis court when his symptoms had began to appear, he finished his coiling action on the court, then uncoiled, and jumped up like nothing had happened. The whole event took about three seconds and appeared to be done with little effort.

"George, are you okay?"

"Oh, yes. I'm glad I didn't break my new glasses,"

he joked.

"Why did you jerk your arm away from me? Do you want me to help you get up now?"

Before he could answer, two men rushed over and started to pick him up without asking. "Wait a minute," I yelled, as they began to lift him.

George said to them, "Why is it that when you're lying down, everyone wants to pick you up? Why don't they let you rest awhile?" Then he added, "You don't want to go in there. Look what happened to me with these new glasses."

The men dropped him back on the ground and skittered away.

When I bent down to see if he was all right, he was laughing.

I ran after the men calling out, "Thank you but you should ask first. He was teasing you." They kept running.

When I returned to George, he was grinning and sitting up waiting for me. How burdensome this must have been for him, yet he handled his weakness with grace and dignity. How strange and tough this thing called living can be.

"That was terrible, George. I should leave you here and do my shopping."

After I retrieved George from the ground, I asked what he wanted to do.

"Let's go to the pub for lunch. Imagine the story I can tell the guys after this one."

That comment made me cranky. How could I get him to understand that he needed assistance walking? His arms were useless, so he couldn't use a walker or a cane. His only options were human assistance, or a wheelchair.

I was tired of dusting him off as I picked him up. I had dusted him more times than I dusted my entire house since he became ill. There was an elephant living in the house with us, and I had to figure out how to introduce George to him. His name: rubber legs. The sensation of falling is fast and enjoyable when you're in the air, free and floating, but it only lasts a short time. Soon people start grabbing at you to pull you up. That isn't half as enjoyable for you or those around you.

A week later I dressed George in his tuxedo to attend our annual class of 1948 West Point New Year's Eve dinner party. Jokingly I asked him, "Why do you torture yourself with these strange dress requirements? Why do you have so many belt loops on your pants?" In my experience, women don't have that many belt loops, but women, of course, have hips to hold up their pants.

As I struggled to tie his black bow tie and engage the tiny buttons on his starched dress shirt, he teased me about my ineptness. I'd tried for months to learn how to tie a four-in-hand knot in his neckties, but I never met his fussy standards. Finally I told him, "When we get to the party, I'll grab one of your classmates, and he can finish dressing you. I can't button these little things. Is that all right with you?"

"Yes, I'm sorry. These are really tiny buttons." He reached over and tried to pat me gently, because he had so little energy. I felt his vulnerability and the struggle it was for him to keep his dignity.

"Are you sure you want to go to this party?" I asked him. "You know what great partiers our friends are. Please tell me when you want to leave."

When we arrived at the party, George said, "Phyl, look at the full moon. It's going to be an exciting evening."

The moonlight was startling and romantic. For a moment or two, I forgot how our lives had changed since that dreadful diagnosis in 2000. I remembered the New Year's Eve class party we had hosted in our home several years back: eating, drinking, dancing, celebrating with these same friends.

George jolted me from my reverie. "Hey, are we going to the party?"

"George, please let me go up the stairs and have one of the guys help us. The temperature's dropped to below freezing, and I'm not comfortable taking you up those icy stairs by myself. I'm wearing an evening gown and high heels, not tennis shoes and workout pants."

"No, we can do this," he said. "I feel fine." Then he gave me his winning smile.

I kept hoping some one else would be arriving soon, and we could go up together so I dragged my feet walking over to his side of my SUV to slide him out, a task in itself. I lowered his backrest and he leaned back enough so I could swing his hips and legs towards me. I brought the backrest erect again, and hugged him under his arms, turning him towards me. His legs came right along with him. Then he stepped down from the car with no problem. I was glad I had the height of the SUV because I would not have been able to pull him out of a lower car.

We headed up the long wrought-iron staircase as I supported George's arm. When George was next to the top platform, I reached up and rang the doorbell. I turned around. George had fallen face down onto the icy platform.

"George, are you okay?" I grabbed him by the seat of his trousers so he wouldn't slide down the stairs.

The door opened, and one of his tall, West Point classmates looked at George, saying, "George, you fighter pilots really know how to party. Are you okay?" By then, another of his husky classmates was standing at the door.

His friends picked him up, dusted him off, took him inside the house, gave him a scotch and water, and the party came alive, even more joyous than before. I gave one classmate George's tie and buttons and said, "Would you please finish dressing George?"

My stubborn mule rider was not to be deterred. George joked, "Yes, we flyboys like to party. But I'm the only one I know who falls into a New Year's Eve party, instead of falling out of the party. Happy New Year!"

When we left his friends wanted to carry him out to the car. Instead we chose to use the garage exit, so our departure was more graceful than our entry. It was an exciting evening.

When I settled him in bed, rubbed and kissed his forehead in the special way he liked, George said, "Don't put lilies on my chest tonight dear, it's too soon." I answered, "But George, you know I'm allergic to lilies. You'll have to let me know when so I can go buy some."

Two days later, after I finished feeding him breakfast—I didn't have conversations with George before he ate—I said to him, "George, we have to talk. You need to help me understand what is going on with you and why you won't accept any assistance when you're walking."

"OK, I'll listen," he said.

"No. I said we have to talk, that means you. I want you to feel in control of what's happening to you, yet I'm fearful for your safety. Help me understand what I can do to make this easier for you and for me."

George was silent for several minutes.

"I haven't hurt myself yet. I know I'm getting worse, but I'm doing it slowly. So I don't think we have to worry."

"I'm not talking about worrying. I want some action on your part to make this more manageable. You are falling more frequently, and your arms can't help you anymore. You need me to assist you. Now tell me how I can do that."

"If I'm going to fall, I can grab onto your arm."

"No," I said. "I don't want you to grab my arm because then you will pull me down with you, and we'll both be in trouble. If I hold on to you, when you start to fall, I can help you but not fall myself. I can let you go down gently if I hang onto you."

"I'd love to have you hanging onto me, but I don't need you to do that. A handicapped person will ask for help when he needs it."

He had asked for help with his dressing, eating, and for me to substitute for him in his tennis group. His safety, his pride, my sanity, and my fatigue were all up for grabs.

This tension between wanting him to have his freedom and independence, and yet to protect his safety was with us all the time, probably more with me than with him. He didn't fear falling. He wasn't ready for a wheelchair in public. To him, being a care receiver must have been as burdensome as being a caregiver. He used his humor to disguise his discomfort, and I found I had adopted a behavior of benign neglect without realizing it.

Two months later George fell again entering the Old Brogue Pub, where we were meeting friends for dinner. It was a cool, dry evening in early March. I was not holding his arm when he tripped. Within the last few days after his shower, I'd noticed that his toes were dragging, and he was raising his feet to avoid tripping. This sudden weakness was foot drop, a serious complication.

With this most recent fall, he wasn't able to curl into a ball because he was projected several feet across the brick patio, his body sprawled, leaving him on his stomach. When I knelt down to talk with him I saw one side of his scraped face. His glasses were still on his face. They were bent, but not broken. I asked if he wanted me to help him, and if he felt sharp pain anywhere.

"Just let me rest a moment," he said.

A few people walked by on their way into the pub. They looked down at him and continued walking.

I wondered if they thought he was drunk. Over the years we had seen a few people stretched out. I took off my coat and covered him, not wanting to pick him up by myself. Fortunately, the people we were meeting came along within a few minutes.

Together we sat him up. I checked his pulse and bones to see that he was intact. His breathing was normal, and he began to use his humor again. "I didn't come all this way for a Bushmills Irish whiskey just to go home without it. Let's eat."

And eat we did. It was like nothing had happened. As we all joked, I fed him dinner, and we carried on like sensible friends, sharing funny stories of our times since we last enjoyed a meal together. But I knew that this was the last time he would fall like this: he would use a wheelchair—or stay home.

When he was settled in the car, he joked, "The next time I fall will be in front of a church, instead of a pub."

"Is that supposed to mean you won't fall again because you don't go to church?"

"Oh, I think you're upset."

"Yes, I am. I love you, but I have to be frank with you. We have to do something about your falling. Independence isn't about going it alone. I'm drained."

Before he could answer, my heart leapt. I saw the glowing eyes of a deer in the reflection of my headlights. I was used to this when we lived in Great Falls, but we'd been gone for a year. George saw the buck, too, and told me to slow my speed without heavy braking. Fortunately, the buck was tucked into the side of the bush on the opposite side of the road. My experience from the past was that he was not likely to jump in front of me if I continued at a slow, even pace—my headlights would keep him hypnotized with a consequent transient lack of motor reactions.

When it worked, I felt like sobbing. This was too much tension for one evening, and I hadn't even had a glass of wine. I felt like I'd been ground into mincemeat.

We finished the ride home in silence. I was afraid to talk because I might say something unkind. But I knew this was the last time we would go out unless he agreed to consider more options for his safety. I made a note to myself to call the ALS Loan Closet, the next day to request a light travel wheelchair. I'd already talked with them the week before. They had a forty-pound chair with a leather strap seat that folded up easily. I planned to leave it in my SUV for when we traveled.

That night, after I settled him, I cried myself to sleep. Watching his body die a little every day, I wanted to die for him. He kept his spirits high and never showed anyone his pain. But he couldn't hide it from me.

I knew I had to make a decision on using the travel wheelchair. It was an ugly, dirty feeling, but necessary to protect his safety. Sometimes tough love is necessary. I hadn't pampered my husband because he had ALS. When he complained about me using handicapped parking spaces, I told him he could sit in the car and enjoy his stubbornness. He would laugh and say, "Get me out of this car, woman. Now."

The next morning while the hospice aide showered

and dressed George, I drove to the ALS chapter and picked up the travel wheelchair. I decided to introduce George to it by having some fun. I told him we were going to the pub for lunch. When I opened the door to the garage, George saw the wheelchair sitting in the driveway. He said, "Phyl, you need to move that thing out of our driveway. Someone must have left it there."

"I did. I drove over to the ALS chapter this morning while Anna was showering and dressing you. I borrowed it from the ALS loan closet."

"Why? We don't need it yet," he said.

"Maybe not, we will have it in the car if we do." Then I added, "Let's play a game. You can push me in this wheelchair down the hill. Then I will push you back up."

George looked at me as though I was crazy. "You want me to do what? I can't push you," he said.

"Well, you can pretend because I'll help you. So let her fly, or as you used to say when flying, 'Wheels up,'" I hollered, as I sat in the seat.

That made him laugh. He placed his hands on the wheelchair handles and away we went. We made it down the slight hill, not very fast as I helped him with my feet making the chair move.

"See, it wasn't so bad, was it." I added, "Now you get in the chair and let me push you."

"Okay, Phyllis, I get the message. We'll use the wheelchair when we go out."

Then he added, "But you're still the craziest person I've ever known, and still the dearest."

I jumped out of the wheelchair and hugged him.

He had his first wheelchair ride going up the hill on a sunny day and then around the neighborhood a few times. We laughed until we couldn't stop. He had saved face and slid graciously into his wheel chair when it was needed. But he never felt wheelchair bound.

Another change. He was able to accept the increasing weakness in himself and be comfortable in his body, just the way it was.

OUR ANGELS OF LIFE

"You're some organizer, Phyl. I'm glad you're on my team."

There is a tension that many terminally ill people embrace: whether to struggle for the possibility of more time through aggressive treatments, or be comforted and call it a day—and a life.

At our February 2002 ALS support group meeting, two speakers came from the local hospice organization to share their program with us. They passed out literature that explained all aspects of the program, reviewed the services they provided, how hospice is paid for as a Medicare program, who is entitled to participate, and how to get an evaluation at home.

Several in our group already had hospice services at home and were still able to attend the support group meetings. They shared how comforting it was for them and their family to have the support of a nurse they could call twenty-four hours a day. In addition, they didn't have to visit a doctor for prescriptions because a physician visited as needed. Several of the men mentioned that hospice services improved their quality of life and that of their wives because of the help that the nursing aides provided with toileting, showering and dressing their husbands.

These features pleased George because he wasn't interested in visiting a doctor's office anymore, except for routine exams with his eye doctor and dentist. Furthermore, what he heard from his ALS friends involved in hospice care convinced him that comfort care would improve his chances to live his life with dignity, while remaining close to those he loved instead of in an institution.

On the way home I asked George about his responses to the meeting and if he was interested in having an evaluation.

"I have no idea how close I am to dying," he said without a pause, "and she said they accept you if you are expected to live six months." He added, "I've already lived more than a year and a half since Dr. Noble told me I had six months to live. What the hell's the magic of six months?"

"There's no magic that I know of, George. Perhaps you didn't hear her say that they re-evaluate you every six months. If you're cured at six months, then you may be released from the program, but you can always re-apply. Their focus is caring, not curing. But there isn't any cure with ALS."

"Well, you decide. Can we afford it? They may help you, but I'm not dead yet," he said. He struggled to reach over and pat me.

"No. It's your decision, not mine, George. Medicare and your military benefit will pay for most of their services."

A week after the support group meeting, George suggested that I call hospice and make an appointment for them to come and do an evaluation of our needs.

A registered nurse arrived March 4, 2002. We sat at our eight-foot oak dining room table where she spread all the forms and materials. George gave me a quizzical look. He told me later that this display gave the appearance of an insurance salesman preparing for the big sale.

She explained hospice services, coverage, and philosophy. An interdisciplinary team, which included a doctor, nurse, social worker, chaplain, nurse's assistants and volunteers, made routine visits to the home to provide comfort care to the patient. Medicines and equipment were provided as needed—for example, a hospital bed and suction machine. Medicare and George's Tricare military benefit would pay for these.

George told her, "Thank you. But don't send a suction machine or a hospital bed to our home. We don't need them."

The nurse continued, saying, "I will make a note of your request. The hospice medical director will review my assessment and determine your eligibility. You'll be notified in a day or two."

As part of her assessment, she asked George about his family. He told her he had one sibling, a sister. He said he hadn't talked with her for years. "My living will states that my sister and my four birth children are prohibited from assisting with my care or any of my health decisions." She looked up at him as though she was surprised at his strong tone and statement.

He quickly added, "And I don't want any social worker telling me I need to make peace with any of them. I like my life the way I live it, and I don't intend to change it."

In addition, he told the nurse he didn't want any chaplain visits. Raised by Episcopalian parents, George was now more comfortable with his knowledge and practice of Buddhism, which he had learned while in Thailand and Japan during his Air Force career.

I wondered why George said this to her. Then I remembered a DVD we had watched less than a month before made by Bill Moyer on death, dying, and saying goodbye. Someone had said on the DVD that hospice workers believed a person should resolve all relationships. They suggested one way to do this was to contact the person with whom you have conflict and say: "Please forgive me; I forgive you. Thank you. I love you. Now I'm going to say goodbye."

When we watched this DVD with friends who had brought it over one evening, the discussion afterwards was noisy. George and I were the only ones who agreed that cleaning up and 'becoming current' in our relationships mattered only with those people who were important in our lives; those who treated us with respect, but not those who disrespected our wishes.

The end of your life was not a time for meeting social requirements, or for social chitchat. George saw it as a time for him to be stress-free as he lived his remaining time, and for him to have a stress-free death. He'd made peace with himself. There was no need to say goodbye.

I had given George the book, *Hard Choices for Loving People*, by Hank Dunn, a former hospice chaplain. George read it often. It sat on his reading table, along with *Tuesdays with Morrie*, by Mitch Albom. We talked about the courage and strength that Hank Dunn had shown by forthrightly addressing very difficult issues and tough decisions, such as artificial feeding, and breathing assisted devices like a ventilator. Dunn wrote that dying without artificial hydration was a compassionate, natural and peaceful way to leave this world.

If he were accepted into the hospice program, George's physician, Dr. Noble, would need to be a partner with hospice to oversee his care, but not make home visits. As part of the Medicare Hospice Benefit, Title XVIII, he would have to co-sign any medications.

I called Dr. Noble. He had been reluctant five months earlier to meet George's requests for no extraordinary measures like a feeding tube, CPR, oxygen, or a ventilator. I now explained to Dr. Noble that George's deterioration had continued, although he continued to walk and enjoy his life. "George still refuses to consider taking Rilutek," I said, "even though you think he should consider it. But he feels the hospice program will help him live a better quality of life and will enable him to die a peaceful death at home."

I held my breath listening to the dreaded silence on the phone line. Finally, Dr. Noble said that he would co-partner with hospice in assuming responsibility for George's care.

"We both thank you," I told him. "I know it isn't an easy decision on your part."

As the hospice nurse was finishing her business, I asked her if I could call the hospice medical director who would be making the decision about George. "If you give me his number, I can call him now." She did.

I called Dr. Hank and gave him all the information he needed. In addition, he was pleased that Dr. Noble would partner with him. He said we'd be accepted immediately without further visits or assessments.

When I told this to George he said, "Good. Why do these people from the same organization have to ask the same questions? These interviews are tiring."

"I'm sorry." I was beginning to feel cranky myself. "But they are doing this for your benefit. They want to be sure we can work together."

The following week a nurse asked George why he decided to join the hospice program. He answered, "My main concern is I'm getting weaker and becoming a burden to my wife." She told me that the hospice team recommended that I take a respite break from his care to avoid burnout. I thanked her for her advice.

For the first few months in the hospice program, they sent a nursing assistant, Anna, three days a week to shower and dress George in the morning. Anna, born in Africa, was tall, sturdy in build and strong, with a most gracious manner, jolly laugh and a wide smile. She and George hit it off immediately. George would tell others and me, "Anna could lift me up by the ears. I do every thing she tells me to." Then he would add, "She's the only one I'll let cut my finger and toe nails. Phyllis gets them bloody."

As George's legs became weaker and he began to have spasms in his thighs, his walking became more unstable. At that point, I asked for Anna five days a week and hospice approved this request. She became the linch-pin of our hospice family. When she had a problem with her tires and had to miss a day, I bought rear tires for her car because she was struggling to survive, living alone.

Also, when we had substitutes, George told me to be sure and take good care of Anna so she didn't get sick. He really liked her. I told him her husband was visiting from Africa. He beamed and said, "Oh, that's all right. You can shower me."

Getting help from hospice meant George and I were able to spend more time together that was not completely focused on George's personal care. The activities of daily living (ADLs) had become the main focus of our life and daily activities. I was worn thin by having to do it all myself, plus teaching and managing the household.

Joy, our hospice nurse, visited twice a month and Dr. Hank, once a month. Joy had a great time with George. I would make a list for Joy of any changes I noted in George's condition and any issues I thought she needed to address.

One time I put on the top of the list: "George fell off the barstool." She started laughing and asked what happened. I told her, "George was watching Wimbledon while I was preparing dinner. He was sitting close by on a bar stool at the granite cook top. He was so excited when

Agassi won that he slide off his seat to the floor." We all had a good laugh. Fortunately, he wasn't hurt.

When she would ask George if he had any issues to discuss before she examined him, he would joke, "Ain't had no satisfaction, ain't had no bowel action." They would sing this like a song, laugh, and address the problem.

Early on I asked Joy for a comfort kit to have in the house in case of need. Instructions were included for each of the drugs: Morphine and Ativan. As a nurse I was familiar with when to use these if George should develop symptoms of anxiety that needed to be treated, or trouble with breathing.

When the word went out among our friends that George was in hospice care, some of our friends stopped calling us. They assumed he was about to die in two weeks, or thereabouts. This was not surprising since studies have shown that a large percentage of people who select hospice care at home die within two weeks of entering the program. It has the reputation of being a death program, not a living program where the mission is to make the quality of life the best possible for the patient and family.

When I became aware that our friends weren't calling, I realized I had to do something to stop this. I created an email file of our friends and wrote a letter in which I told them that even though George had decided to enter the hospice program at home, his condition hadn't changed. He was still eager to do things with his friends. Next, I sent funny postcards to people whose email addresses I didn't have. Lastly, I used the telephone for those I had missed.

The email and telephone responses were fast. Our friends were thrilled to learn that George wasn't on his way out of this world. Their knowledge of hospice was similar to most folks: this meant the end was very close. It wasn't. George lived over a year in hospice care.

George grinned when I told him what I had done. "You're some organizer, Phyl." He added, "I'm glad you're on my team."

I hugged him and joked, "Don't forget that." The slightest human contact brought immediate joy to both of us.

FINDING FUN IN CRAZY PLACES

"What did you do to my drink this time, woman? It's thick and stinky, again."

"Here's how we play it," I told George one evening when he was drinking his hot toddy and I was fixing dinner. I had decided to create a new ritual and game called 'humor hunt,' where we would dig for humor in our day like a dog digs for bones.

"We meet here at around 5:00 p.m. I'll fix our drinks, and we can sit and share the funny things that happened in our day. You'll get to go first."

"Well, that's a first," he said, his mischievous spirit coming alive again.

I was surprised the next evening when he started the game by giving me his car keys. "You're now my designated driver. No more wine for you."

"What, you mean you've decided to stop driving?" Acting surprised, I was relieved because I wouldn't ride with him. He used to tell me, "Phyl, if you take off the emergency brake, then I can drive. I have to get out of the car to take it off, and it takes a while to get back in."

"Why do you put it on?" I asked him. "You only drive to the Village. There are no hills to park on."

I wasn't sure if he was joking. But I knew that it was a tough decision for him to give up the 'stick,' a common expression, particularly among men, of the 1940s, associated mainly with guns, cars, and sports, particularly polo. For George, a marksman as a teenager, a polo player, and a command pilot in Vietnam, the stick was all-important. He'd learned to drive using a stick shift in 1940 and he continued to use one in his current car.

I had felt conflicted in how to help him in this difficult decision and accepted that I couldn't really help, except to tell him I would take him anywhere he wanted to go, anytime. But I had called Bill, our insurance agent, to advise me on how to deal with this situation. He said, "George will know, as a pilot, when it's time to stop. He won't hurt anyone. But I'll increase your insurance," he said, and offered to come over in the evenings to visit with George so I could get some time away. Bill's mother had died of Lou Gehrig's disease, so he understood our situation. I thanked him and asked if there was any night that he preferred. George liked him, and that would give me time to do some errands.

Later, when I drove with George sitting in the passenger seat, he put a brown paper bag over his head so he didn't have to watch me drive.

"Get that bag off your head. The police will stop us and think I'm kidnapping you."

"You can kidnap me any time," he teased.

Dressing George, feeding him, and all the normal activities of daily living took on a new focus because he needed more help each day. The lifestyle changes forced on us because of this disease required new sources of fun to continue nurturing our husband-wife connection.

George was a meticulous dresser. His shoes were always polished, his socks and ties matched, his shirts were starched to his liking and his pants held perfect creases. When he undressed, he hung his trousers exactly to match the seams. His closet was the neatest in the household.

When I had trouble getting his tee shirt over his head and jerked him around a bit, he'd say during our 'humor hunt' fun time "Hey, woman, how would you like it if I snapped your brassiere like you did with my shirt this morning?"

The nightly humor hunt became our special bonding ritual.

I had to learn to dress him in the same sequence he used himself. No other way would do. The socks and shoes went on before the pants and shirt.

"Why?" I asked.

"I put my socks and shoes on before my pants and shirt so that I don't choke myself on my shirt collar and necktie bending over to tie my shoes," he explained.

Choosing not to argue with him by reminding him that I was doing the bending over and tying, I did what he asked and concentrated on other tasks like learning how to tie a four-in-hand necktie. I was never able to do it to his satisfaction. I carried his ties with me in my purse when we went out. It had become a joke when I'd pull them out and ask our friends, "Would you please finish dressing George?"

George loved to tell stories about his wife to anyone who would listen. I'd go up behind him, smile at him, hug him and whisper in his ear, "ABC, George." This was my shorthand message for 'Avoid Boring Conversations,' or talking about your wife. One night he had everybody laughing when he told them this fish story.

"When I was sitting on the bar stool at the cook-top island in our kitchen, Phyllis was cooking one of my favorite fish dishes—sautéed tilapia with fresh garlic in olive oil.

"She prepared the pan for the fish and began making my hot toddy. As she mixed my drink, I could see that the Bushmills wasn't blending with the sugar, lemon juice and water. She continued to stir it vigorously. I wondered if she thought the sugar hadn't dissolved—a trick a tired mind can play on you.

"She placed my drink with my long, glass straw next to me on the counter and went back to see how the fish was doing. It was doing strange things as well. It was flipping around, jumping up and down in the pan.

"'What did you do to my drink this time, woman?' I asked her. 'It's thick and stinky, again.'

"As she turned to answer me, I saw the tilapia in the frying pan dancing like they were drunk, flying up in the air. Evidently she'd put the whiskey in the frying pan with the fish, and it became poached tilapia. It was good.

"She'd put the olive oil in my hot toddy. It was awful.

"She made me a fresh hot toddy and we enjoyed Bushmills poached tilapia, a new recipe."

Another way he teased me when I showered him and dried him was to talk about things he wanted to do that day. As I dried his ears by putting my fingers with the end of the towel in his ears, I asked him a question or answered his. Then he would holler at me, "Phyllis, how do you expect me to hear you when you block my ears by sticking your fingers in my ears. I'm not deaf you know."

"You are too. You're deaf from all those years of flying fighters. I'm probably just tired and acting stupidly, but standing this close to me, you should be able to read my lips," I said, and wacked him on his disappearing butt.

Because he drifted off as we were sharing stories in our humor hunt, I realized that George's strength was declining so I developed a new ritual for him: the afternoon nap. When I suggested this to him, he protested.

"Sleep in the middle of the day? I don't think so."

"If you want to keep up your schedule of dinner with friends, you'll enjoy it more if you have a nap in the afternoon. That way you can save your strength and feed yourself some of the time when we're out."

We scheduled naptime each day. He teased me by coming up, trying to stretch like a cat, rubbing against me, and purring in my ear so I would help him into bed. He couldn't put his arms or paws up like a cat but he tried to imitate one. He wanted to be petted and rubbed once he lay down, too. I teased him and said, "Petting time?"

He answered, "Not any more. Wish I could."

We learned that one of the pivotal moments in a loving relationship happens when a loved one comes to understand that vulnerability is what binds us to each other, and love happens because of that, not in spite of it. We learned that being present to each other was what really mattered.

Another ritual that I created was for George to reach out to his friends who called him. He didn't like talking on the phone, maybe because his hearing was damaged. Thus, he let the recording machine take the calls while I was away.

"You need to get involved doing something every day that takes you out of yourself and keeps you connected with your friends," I told him. "They want to hear from you, not me. They're trying to tell you they are here to help. I'm tired of telling everyone about you. You can help me with this."

"Men don't talk about their illnesses, or get involved in each other's business like you women do," he said.

"What a loss for you guys. Think of all the fun you miss talking with each other. We talk with our friends because we care about them, and we want to help each other. You men always talk about issues, which keeps you distant from your friends."

"That's what you women are for—to help us men," he said as he sat up grinning, waiting to see if I was going to throw something at him.

I was about to pick up a shoe and send it in his direction when I looked at him and said to myself, *George is either jerking me around, or teasing me with serious intent.*

Whatever it was, I didn't like it. I was over the limit with fatigue because of caring for all his daily physical needs, taking telephone calls which he wouldn't take, and getting him to visit friends and support groups. He wanted me there with him most of the time, but he feared being a burden. That tension created some sad moments for him because he knew the journey was tough as hell for both of us.

I decided he had to put out more effort. We could survive the ugly parts of the illness only if we helped each other.

"Listen, you, I'll make a list of the friends you used to have lunch, discuss investing, or play tennis with. I think you should call one of them every couple of days and talk with him."

"About what?" He added, "They're okay or someone would let me know."

"That's the point. You just wait for someone to give you the news. You need to reach out and connect with your friends. First, you might say, "It's been awhile since we've talked. How are things going with you? I heard of an interesting company for investing that might interest you—something like that."

I added, "What did you talk about before you became ill?"

He put his head down on his chest and after awhile he said, "I can't dial or hold the phone long enough to do that." His voice was subdued and muffled.

Then I realized that part of his reluctance to call his friends was a consequence of this disease devouring his body. He had lost confidence to talk with his friends. He may have been embarrassed to tell me of his increasing vulnerability.

I ran over and hugged him.

After we shared a large glass of orange juice, I said to him, "How about I buy a speaker phone and put it on your desk? I'll enter the numbers of your friends, and all you'll need to do is press a button. Will that work for you?"

"OK, let's try it. I know better than to fight with you, Phyl, because you'll do it anyway." He tried to give me a slight pinch on my fanny.

"When I come home from work, you can tell me some juicy news that I can pass on to the wives. You know how we love to gossip. This might be fun. We could start a riot."

After I set up the phone on his desk, when I came home George would tease me. "So who did *you* call today? What's the latest news?" He smirked like a fox—daring me to ask him the same thing.

As it turned out, George began to connect with old

friends he had missed seeing because of his illness. His treasured tennis buddy from Army Navy Club had moved to Florida with his terminally ill wife to be close to their family. I would hear gales of laughter coming from the bedroom when he and George spoke every week. Also, I located his long-time secretary who lived in Florida. They talked and renewed their long-time friendship each week.

A new world of connections opened for George that provided him company and loving experiences. He thanked me for being so gentle in pushing him. "Well, I wouldn't say I was gentle," I told him, and tucked him in for a good nap.

Because our new town house was a plumbing nightmare, funny things continued to happen to us as we struggled to live with this terminal disease. Over many months, at varying times, all four floors received periodic baths on ceilings, carpeting, walls, and floors.

There were times when we had water coming from around the ceiling sprinklers, coming from the kitchen ceiling, coming from the washing machine hoses, bathroom fixtures; we had water draining outside the house from an emergency valve associated with the water heater on the fourth floor, and from the drainage pan underneath the water heater. Each time they repaired a problem, another problem surfaced.

One afternoon when we came home from a lovely

brunch on Father's Day at the 1763 Inn, I shrieked in horror at the sight of the living room ceiling partially collapsed on our large coffee table and new Karastan wool rugs, as water continued to drip from the ceiling.

But the biggest problem was in our bathroom where I showered George in the walk-in shower. The drain in this shower intermittently backed up as workers repaired other plumbing problems. As a consequence, we had soaked carpeting and walls that needed to be replaced in the hallway leading from the bathroom to the bedroom and in the closets alongside the long hallway. Clothes were soaked and ceilings were sinking. We had no way to give George a shower without this walk-in arrangement which also had a tiled seat where he could rest and have the comforting warm water flow over his back and legs for several minutes.

After obtaining the services of an attorney, we moved to a hotel for a month while the builder rebuilt our plumbing system and replaced carpeting and walls. I also brought in an inspector certified by the Environmental Protection Agency (EPA) to check for mold in the structure, which he found. This meant the house had to be closed after all the repair work was completed while mold killer was blown throughout. The house was sealed for several days.

Coincidentally, we had close friends arriving from London who wanted to see George while he was still up for guests and having fun. We took them to the hotel with us, at the builders' expense. They were appalled that this could happen in America.

Our hospice aide, Anna, came to the hotel to care for him while I worked with the contractors at our town house to supervise and be sure they did it right this time. The day we returned home we were excited for George to have a good shower, which hadn't been possible in the cramped hotel shower.

At dinner, we celebrated with wine and Bushmills and joked about our humor hunt for the evening as we ate dinner once again in our new home. It felt so good to us. After a pleasant, relaxed evening together, we went upstairs to get ready for bed.

George eagerly walked into his newly repaired shower. When I had him soaped up and was lathering shampoo over his hair, I thought I felt water climbing up my legs to my knees. But I dismissed that feeling because I knew they had fixed our shower.

"Phyllis, why is the water rising in the shower?" George asked. I looked down and noticed the shower drain wasn't working, and the water was rising fast in the shower stall. Soon, the bathroom floor was flooded again, as I tried to rinse off the soap and shampoo from George. I was soaked throughout. My clothes stuck to my body, and my hair clung to my head in clumps.

The new carpeting was soaked again and would need to be replaced.

We looked at each other and burst into raucous laughter at the absurdity of the situation. I think we laughed to keep from crying. I said to George, "Remember what Victor Hugo said. 'Laughter is the sun that drives winter from the human face.'" We were glowing with sunshine, soap, and shampoo.

I took George back to the hotel the next morning so they could repair the shower again, and replace soggy carpeting and damaged woodwork.

The builder determined later that the person who put in the new tile in the shower had failed to protect the excess plaster from falling into the water drain. The shower drain became clogged because it was full of old plaster. No one had tested the drain to see if it worked.

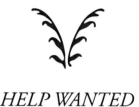

HELP WANTED

"What are you trying to do to me, woman? Kill me?"

When the hospice team finished their evaluation of George for their program, they all agreed I needed a break from being the only person meeting all of George's needs. They suggested I call a home care agency and bring in someone three times a week. Also, they noted that George wasn't able to use the elevator by himself. Then they pointed out two dangers: our big dog, Nicky, could trip George; and George wasn't stable on the stairs because he couldn't use his arms to hang onto the railings. We were fast approaching the time when it wasn't safe to leave George alone.

After several nights of little sleep for both of us, I decided to fix us an early dinner and talk with George about my plan to call a home care agency. As a very private man, he didn't want strangers in our home. I didn't either. It felt like an invasion of our carefully protected privacy.

But a stranger had come into our home uninvited well over a year ago: Lou Gehrig. Most visitors smell after three days. Lou Gehrig's disease really smelled after a year. We had to accept that this stranger wasn't going to leave, so I had to get some assistance. Otherwise, my tiredness could accidentally harm George. He worried about becoming a burden to me; yet, he wanted me with him all the time. I didn't want strangers either, but I was becoming a stranger to him and to myself. I had begun doing dumb things.

A few months earlier, I had forgotten to zip his trousers before we began our escorted Christmas Tour of the Biltmore Museum in North Carolina. As we stood, with me carrying my sleeping seven-month-old granddaughter, I scrambled around in my mind for a place to go to zip his fly. The crowded festive lobby sported two Christmas trees decorated with antique ornaments. Boxes tied with velvet ribbons waited beneath the trees, and Christmas music filled the air.

I thought, *Do we go to the women's or the men's room, or find a potted plant to hide behind?* I decided we should do it in the car.

"I think we have to do it in the car," I whispered to George.

"Phyl, I can't do it in the car anymore," he said loud enough that everyone could hear. Some people gasped, others howled. My answer to him, "Honey, you never could," halted the tour, as laughter erupted from every direction. The noise woke my granddaughter, who kicked me in the stomach as she grabbed my long hair to climb up on my shoulder. We skittered away to the car like naughty penguins.

Laughing as I remembered this incident, I went upstairs and found George struggling with his computer. I decided to tell him my plan. "How about an early dinner, some conversation, and an early to bed for both of us?"

"Sounds good to me. What's for dinner?" he said.

"How about some of your favorites: citrus salmon with garlicky greens, sautéed summer squash, French bread, chocolate ice cream sundae, and your special orange Gatorade?"

"Okay, but don't forget my Bushmills hot toddy before dinner. And I can't chew the nuts on the sundae anymore."

"Fine, then let's turn off your computer and take the elevator downstairs." I moved over to help him. This small task was becoming more difficult for him.

Preparing our meal, I watched George out of the corner of my eye as he sat on the bar stool at our kitchen island drinking his Bushmills and being near me. I was careful not to act as his nurse, but my radar was always turned to where he was. At the same time, I tried not to hover over him like a hawk.

But he wouldn't change his pattern of where and how he sat. He told me he had learned to sit with his legs and feet tucked around the back of the stool to prevent him from slipping. He was engrossed watching tennis, our favorite sport during our marriage.

As we began our dinner with more tennis, we were happy. George still struggled to feed himself by bending down from his waist and curving his arm around his plate, barely hanging on to his fork. He was able to drink liquids from a long straw that I put in a tall glass. He was quiet as he drank, ate, and watched tennis.

I looked over at his face to see if he was enjoying his dinner and drink, but I found only a contorted look as he tried to use the straw to drink his Gatorade. I wondered why he looked so strange. Was his illness progressing so fast that he couldn't draw liquid through the straw?

After he'd made three futile attempts to drink the orange Gatorade, George said, "What are you trying to do to me, woman? Kill me?"

Surprised, I thought he was joking.

"Hell, what am I drinking?" he said.

"You're drinking Gatorade," I said.

"It tastes like glue, and it won't move in my glass."

All of a sudden, we both burst out laughing. I couldn't stop.

"You're on overload, woman. You gave me Nicky's Citrucel for his bowel movements. I'm not a dog. I don't need any help going to the bathroom."

I realized he was right. The Citrucel had the same color and granules as the Gatorade.

At our feet, Nicky slurped up his food thoroughly soaked in Gatorade. His beautiful white chest was yellow-orange and sticky. With the contrast of his heavy, long, black hair and the orange Gatorade, he looked like a Halloween character, surrounded by a floor covered with orange splatters of Gatorade.

He looked up grateful.

At that point, I was too tired to discuss anything

serious, since we both kept laughing as Nicky entertained us. I took Nicky outside and gave him a spit bath with the hose. We were both soaked when we came back in. George just shook his head at us and turned to watch more tennis.

A few days later our friend, Dianne, came over to learn about investing in the financial markets. We had been doing this for several months with other friends who had moved away. But George liked to teach and talk about investments anytime. He had returned to study for a Doctorate in International Finance after he retired from the Air Force in 1973 and had taught finance at several universities before he retired. More importantly, George had learned investing at the feet of his father who had a seat on Wall Street up into his seventies. Dianne and I were pleased he would teach us.

George and I kept separate investment portfolios because our investment strategies differed. George's strategy was more conservative than mine because he didn't include social variables in his models, variables that I thought, as a sociologist, were important. We always enjoyed discussing our investments, and at the end of the year we'd compare our results to see who came out better. Most of the time, I did, so he expanded his models and variables. We teased and pushed each other. It was great fun.

Dianne and I took George downstairs in the elevator to set up the video for class. I brought drinks and a small snack to accompany our two-hour adventure. George could sip his drink by himself through his long straw on a side table. He was always prepared with typed up notes and a video to illustrate the main points.

Dianne and I listened while he explained the concepts with examples. He asked if we had any questions. I didn't, but Dianne did. Then he asked me to please turn on the fifty-minute video.

Eager to sink into one of our new Jessica Charles' Bedford Swivel Rockers to watch the video, I slid onto the high, tufted backrest of the chair, my arms on the quilted armrests, and put my feet on the matching ottoman. Promptly, I went to sleep. Soon I thought I could hear myself snore, but even that racket didn't wake me up. When the video was finished, Dianne woke me. I was embarrassed, but nobody cared that I had slept.

After that I decided I had to get some help or I might accidentally harm my husband and myself. But it got worse before I acted. The next morning as I backed out of the driveway, my mind was on George's difficult night. A urinary infection had him up to the bathroom many times—with my help. Although a low-grade prostate cancer had been treated with radiation in 1997, he continued to have an enlarged prostate that often made it difficult for him to pee. Sometimes this caused an infection. I was on my way to the pharmacy to pick up his antibiotics while our hospice nursing assistant was there to shower and dress him.

When I heard the ugly crunch and scraping of

metal against metal, I jammed on my brakes. Only then did I realize I hadn't bothered to check my rearview mirror for cars. No one ever parked in our townhouse driveway, but I had plowed into Anna's car. She'd never parked there before, but I had told her if she couldn't find a parking place to use the driveway.

Fortunately, more damage was done to my SUV than hers. When she left that morning, I showed her what I had done and said I'd pay to have it repaired. She laughed and told me I needed to bring in more assistants.

Harvey, Dianne's husband, repaired the slight damage done to Anna's car, putting in a new back-up light on one side.

A few days later George saw the dent in my car on the right fender above the tire. I had tried to keep him from seeing it, but he was still checking out what was going on. He laughed and said, "What did you do now?"

I lied to him. Sometimes I woke up and thought I'd lost all my senses.

A week later I talked with George and said I was going to call a home health care agency for an additional assistant to work four hours a day twice a week. "If this works out to give us more quality time together, then we can increase the hours."

"So what's this person going to do? Just sit here? And where will you be?"

"I'm supposed to return to teaching part-time soon.

The nurse's aide would be with you to feed you dinner and prepare you for bed while I'm gone. So when I come home, we can relax together before bedtime," I said.

"I don't want someone here when you're gone. I don't want to be left alone with strangers in my home."

"I know that, but I need some time to do errands. How about trying this. I will train one or two workers over a two or three week period. That way you can decide whether you feel comfortable with the person. If you don't, we can try something else, like calling our friends to come while I teach."

"We can try it," he said. His voice was not convincing, and he turned away from me.

My legs felt like jelly. His vulnerability was anguishing to me. He had to rely on others to treat and care for him in a fair, open, and honest way. He had been a decorated military officer, then a professor, and now he was reduced to being cared for like a baby. I could only imagine the courage and strength that required. I also understood that my presence was the dearest thing I could share with him.

Yet, I couldn't be there all the time. I had to walk away from my role in his illness and be competent in another way, such as in my teaching. On the other side, George had taught me to slow down in our daily relationships. He couldn't chew any faster, so I had to feed him at a slower pace or he would choke. I couldn't dress him any faster or put on his socks and shoes any faster since he couldn't help me. Slowdown was necessary for both of us if we were going to be able to 'let go'. Letting go was part of our story, an important part.

I called a home health agency, interviewed applicants, and trained them. After training one woman for two weeks in his presence, the first day I prepared to leave for my classes, George said, "You're not going to leave me with her, are you?" I wanted to either belt him one, or drop to the floor and cry.

"Yes, I am," I said. "And I expect you to have a good time and tell me all about your new adventures when I get home." Then I cried all the way to school.

In the following months, I had to fire two of the women I'd trained when they didn't do their jobs. One night, I came home from school, kissed George, and nearly fell over.

"You smell like ammonia—like you just ate a dead cat! Did she brush your teeth?"

"No, she told me she doesn't brush teeth."

I ran downstairs before the nursing aide prepared to leave and asked her why she hadn't brushed his teeth when I had shown her how to use the electric toothbrush and to do it. She replied, "I don't like to do that. It's nasty."

I answered, "And so are you. Get out, and don't come back. I'll call the agency and tell them why." After she left, I slammed the front door. Poor George. Having to deal with this when he was so ill. I felt ashamed for leaving him.

George declined to let the aides feed him the dinner I had prepared for him. He told them he would wait for his wife to eat. He sat at the head of the stairs where he could hear the garage door rise. That's how he knew I was home.

Two days before Christmas, I came home early and found George bent over, with his face down on his computer. That aide sat beside him, laughing and talking on her cell phone in a foreign language. She continued talking when I came into the room. My heart nearly burst with anger and pain as I grabbed a hold of the chair she was sitting on. Trembling with rage, I had to fight the urge to harm her. Then I flipped, and trying not to shout said, "You're fired. Get Out! I've warned you four times about this. I'll call the agency and tell them you're not coming back here."

"But Christmas is almost here," she said.

"Get out before I throw you out." I gained control of myself, ran back to my husband, and dug his face out of his computer.

I decided it was time to stop teaching. I would find other ways to get help.

When we returned from our annual Christmas vacation in the Virginia mountains with our family, I asked George to help me develop a plan whereby we could accept help from our friends who continued to ask what they could do to help us. "What do they want to do?" he asked.

"They've offered to drive you to your monthly book club, take you to lunch, visit you at home so I can get out and do errands more quickly." I gave him other ideas like take him to get a haircut, help him with his computer.

"Where will you be?" he asked.

"I'll probably take a nap while you're gone," I joked. "I have plenty to do that I have neglected because I run out of energy and time, like clean the house, shop, pay bills."

"Okay, we can try it. But it sounds strange to me."

"I need you to tell me how to use the Excel program on my laptop so I can organize a plan. I can put in the names of our friends who have offered to help and what they want to do." I added, "It would help me if you would tell me who you want on the list, and what you would be comfortable having them help you with."

Using Excel software on my Apple laptop computer, I listed friends who lived in the local community, friends who lived within an easy commuting distance, including phone numbers, and email addresses. In another column I listed the type of resources they might be able to provide: rides, time to relieve me, meals, and other categories. I enlarged the matrix to include the types of help I needed, times I preferred, and other options, and emergency numbers.

During my childhood in foster homes and an orphanage, and later as a Charge Nurse, and Chair of a university department, I had learned how to organize to my benefit. These skills taught me how to survive.

When I worked to match people on the matrix, I was careful to spread out the jobs so as not to tire them. Another category on the matrix was the date the person was called and when I assigned that person a job. I included a substitute who would be available if there was a need.

Next, I created an email list and sent it to the people on the list and asked for their permission to be on the list and additional comments. They answered quickly with every positive way they could help us and enjoy these difficult times with us. I was overwhelmed by their generosity and kindness.

I printed a copy of the matrix and kept it by each of the four telephones in the house. It was a winner.

I reminded myself that providing good care for George depended on providing good care for me, first.

A BIDET TODAY KEEPS THE WIFE AWAY

"There are only two rules. You don't wash your feet in it, and only one person at a time can enjoy it."

"Good grief, woman, what is that contraption on the toilet seat with those red and green blinking lights?" George asked me when he came into my office. We had just returned from having lunch with friends.

"It's a bidet, George. Today is happy bidet day. You told me that when you travelled in the military, every bathroom in France had one. You guys used to joke about the racy French bathrooms."

"OK, but where did it come from and what it's doing in our bathroom?"

"It's a present for you," I answered, somewhat miffed at his seemingly stupid and ungrateful questions. "You mentioned a week ago that you were having more difficulty wiping your bum because your arms are getting weaker. This is your 'bum helper.' I know you don't want me to wipe your butt, and the bidet is happy to do all the work for you. Harvey put it in while we were at lunch."

"All right. Now, please, just tell me how it works."

"I will if you smarten up and act more appreciative of what's being done to help you to maintain your glorious independence. I've wiped enough butts as a nurse, and I'm not wiping yours if there's technology to do it. A bidet today keeps your wife away."

"Really? Let's go upstairs and you can demonstrate how to use it," he teased.

We laughed, because the latest addition to his dressing routine was wearing sweatpants during the day since he couldn't work the belt or zipper on his regular trousers. When we went out with friends, he had to limit his fluid intake because there were no unisex bathrooms where I could help him pee. We joked about whether we would cause more panic if I took him to a family restroom, the women's room, or the men's room.

"Here's the card that gives you all the operating instructions," I said. "Read it and then I'll show you how to work the two buttons that wash and dry your bum. Your right arm will rest comfortably over the control panel and I'll show you how to manage it. Then you're on your own."

"OK, but I really have to pee now. Can we use one of the other bathrooms?"

"That's up to you, but the bidet doesn't affect your peeing. It's just like a regular toilet seat, except that it's heated. It has a panel of water controls on the right side. Just lift up the toilet seat to pee like you always do."

"Well, since you have to pull down my pants so I can pee, let's go look at the bidet." He added, "You must be tired of doing this so many times a day."

I thought to myself, *Even impossible things become routine if you repeat them often enough.*

"So who's counting?" I said. "I'd rather do it than clean up a mess."

"Well, I'm tired of it, and you have to do it at least eight to ten times a day."

"Get over it, please," I answered.

We were comfortable communicating non-verbally. I knew when to pull down his pants and when to pull them up without either of us talking about it, unless he was in a randy mood.

We went upstairs to our master bedroom where I took off his jacket so he would be comfortable on the bidet seat. Then we entered the enclosed toilet closet in our master bathroom, and I pulled down his pants so he could pee. I left George for a minute and entered the larger bathroom that contained the tiled glass shower with a built-in seat for him to use during his shower.

I sat down on the edge of my Jacuzzi bathtub, where I sank every night with a book, a glass of red wine, and bubble bath. I lost myself in the sweet scent of lavender and bubbles until I was only a small pair of eyes peeking through bubbles. Although I was always listening for his call, I tried to relax after he was in bed.

These days, much of our life took place in this bathroom: toileting, bathing, dressing, answering the telephone—and more. What health professionals call the activities of daily living (ADLs) ruled our life. Thank goodness, the bathroom was roomy enough for a wheelchair and all of George's paraphernalia.

As I looked across the room into the mirror that covered the entire wall, I caught a glimpse of my face. Realizing that my hair looked like I'd combed it with a broom, the tears slid from my eyes. Sometimes when I took him to the bathroom, I didn't remember which one of us had to pee.

George tried to be brave, not showing any frustration or despair as his physical condition deteriorated beyond his control. I turned on his Bose music system with his favorite CDs of New Orleans jazz.

After I heard the toilet flush, I went to the toilet to show him how to work the bidet. "How many times a day do you get to look at my genitals? Beautiful, aren't they?" he said laughing heartily. Then he added, "Hurry up woman. I don't have all day."

"You're still a randy old fighter pilot," I said. "They are beautiful, but I'd rather look at your face, thank you. Turn around, please, and sit on the bidet seat. Let's review the instructions before I pull your sweatpants up over your legs, in case you get squirted by mistake."

I showed him how to rest his right arm on the attached control panel that contained the buttons to activate the water hoses. "Press the BACK button to start the back wash that cleans your butt with warm water for two minutes. If you want to repeat the wash, press the button again. Any time you want to stop the wash or dry actions, press the STOP button. Just give it a light touch."

"Have you tried it yet?" he asked. "I think you

should try it first."

"No, I haven't. Now go ahead and press the BACK button. It's your toy, and you get to use it first. It should spray warm water around your bum area. The bidet washes your bum after you poop."

I could see the mischief gathering in his sapphire blue eyes, so I continued quickly, "Now let me show you the DRY button which is behind the BACK button. Look at it so you'll know where to press it." I added, "It dries for two minutes but if you need more, hit it again."

"Wow, this seat is warm and cozy. I'm going to try this tonight after you shower me."

"I think you might try it before I shower you. That way your bum will be spanking clean."

The bidet, in addition to adding humor to our lives, improved my husband's quality of life. As a nurse I'd learned that running warm water on your butt relaxes the abdominal muscles. When he had difficulty with stuck BMs, he'd run the warm water over his anus, which helped his sphincter relax, stimulating action and satisfaction. I told him there were no bowel movements in Heaven, and that's why all men wanted to go there.

Also, the seat warmer encouraged him to move his bowels because to warm up a seat with a cold body takes quite a while. A cold seat makes your anus pucker, clamp down, and close.

Despite his weakened arms, the bidet became a lifesaver for him by providing him both privacy and dignity at a time when these were sliding away, despite my efforts to preserve them.

In his usual approach to our new life, George found a way to make the bidet story humorous. He went on the Internet and found bidet jokes that he shared with his friends in the ALS support group, with the hospice workers, and with others who were curious about his new toy. He told them, "Bidet means 'pony' in French. So you position yourself on the toilet seat like it was a pony." He added, "Our grandchildren own horses and they jump on and off the bidet as they flood the bathroom. They have a great time."

I kept wine in the bathroom for our curious friends who enjoyed bidet humor, wine and conversation when they visited. They asked him, "What is the proper etiquette for using the bidet?" George told them, "There is no etiquette for using it. There are only two rules. You don't wash your feet in it, and only one person at a time can enjoy it."

There were fits of giggling, ribald humor, and general hilarity because a bidet in every home is not a part of our bidet-less society. For some, there was trepidation about what was the correct way to use one. They peeked at it and asked questions, acting as if it were a rocket about to take off.

The most often asked questions were, "What holds it on the toilet? How do you operate it?" and "Is it hot?" I handed them the operating instructions card that hung on the wall next to it. After they read it, George said, "This is easy. Two presses and you're done with a sparkling bum." One doctor said he was going to buy one for his wife.

George joked with anyone who would listen to

him, "Cleaning with water is much more comforting than using toilet paper. I'd never go back to toilet paper." Then someone would shriek, "What! You don't use toilet paper?"

George said, "No. The bidet saves trees."

The bidet was George's buddy until his death.

And mine, too.

WAITING

"Phyllis, you are the craziest person I know, and the dearest!"

On any given day, after months of caring for someone, you find yourself not knowing what day it is, and wrestling with your own spiritual loneliness. Suddenly you want to make the dying hurry up so you don't have to constantly witness the pain. It was hard to watch George struggle so valiantly, to watch death happen every day, and to not yearn to die with him or for him.

One evening after dinner, when we'd finished watching the Wimbledon tennis finals in the family room, George grew quiet. Feeling a little weepy, we joked about the fact that I still played for him in his men's group, using his god-awful heavy racket, so that he could still be 'on the court' with his friends.

As I finished cleaning up the kitchen, I asked him to tell me about his greatest frustrations so far on this journey. He didn't answer. I wondered if he'd heard me since he didn't wear his hearing aid anymore. Perhaps he was asleep.

Finally, he said, "I'm tired of waiting."

"Waiting? For what?" I asked.

"That could take all night. There's just too much to say."

"Well, I have all night. Let's talk about it."

I prepared his hot toddy, and a glass of pinot noir for me. Then we talked for more than an hour, with our eyes tearing up in pain and tender laughter. It was the first time George shared what it meant to him to wait for each moment of living—and dying. This began many hours of sharing. Over many months, these were some of the things that George told me were hard or meant a lot to him:

"When I wake up, I wait to see if my eyes are getting worse. They are.

"I wait to feel if I can move my head, my arms or legs. Each day I can move less.

"I wait to see if I can still whistle. I worry that if I lose my whistle, I won't be able to call you when I need you. I love our joke that this is the only time I can whistle for you without getting a shoe thrown at me.

"I wait for your smile.

"I wait for you to get me out of bed into the wheelchair, lift me out of the wheelchair onto the bidet, and close the bathroom door and let me sit alone for a few minutes. I love that you tell me it's time for bowel movements with Beethoven, and then you turn on the Bose music system. You always say that you'd love to smell some sweet-smelling shit when you return.

"I wait for you to get me back into my wheelchair, wash my hands and face, and take me downstairs.

"I wait for you to turn on the news and feed me my favorite breakfast of old-fashioned oatmeal, orange juice, toast, and strong coffee. And I enjoy watching the news while you clean up the kitchen.

"I wait for you to take me upstairs after breakfast and prepare me for my shower. When you lift me from the wheelchair, undress me and sit me onto the shower chair, it's so great that you talk to me—hug and hold me. We play around as I give you orders: 'Hurry up, woman. I don't have all day.' And then I add, 'Hey, slow down, woman, this is kinda fun—just like our honeymoon.' We play like the baby pandas at the Washington Zoo.

"I wait for you to rub shampoo on my head, massage my scalp as you wash my hair. Then you run the shower water over my body and let me relax with the warm water running over my back and legs. That feels so good! You get wetter than I do, so I encourage you to wear your bikini the next time, or maybe nothing at all. Then you smack me on my disappearing butt, and call me a randy old fighter pilot.

"I wait for you to dry and dress me after I tell you what I want to wear. You sit on the floor. It's so hard for you to put on my socks and shoes because I can't push with my feet, or hold my feet or legs up. But you won't let me wear slippers during the day and feel like a prisoner of war, deprived of the dignity of socks and shoes. It means so much to me that you help me keep my dignity.

"I wait while you rub talcum powder on my face before you use my electric razor to shave off the chin stubble. I watch you in the mirror and see my facial bones are melting away. Sometimes I tease you when you brush my teeth with the electric toothbrush, nibbling on your fingers or clamping down on the toothbrush. We always laugh a lot. Oh how I love our laughter.

"I wait while you get me seated in front of my computer, which you have to help me use now, because my hands aren't agile enough. We're a funny-looking pair. You don't know how to work the computer, and although I know how, I can't, because my hands don't work any more.

"I wait for our grandchildren to visit, climb up in my bed, feed me lunch, comb my hair, and brush my teeth. I love it when they scold me: 'Grandpa George, you can't go out and play unless you eat all your lunch.' Then you get me out of bed so the girls can walk me around the room to the elevator using the makeshift toy crutches they've made for me with pieces of wooden tinker toys that they connected together. You grab me hard from behind by my pajama bottoms to hold me up, while the girls place a crutch under each arm and hold my hands, as we parade to the elevator. I'm determined not to fall in front of them.

"I wait for Joy, our hospice nurse, and Dr. Hank, to come for their visits. They do their usual examinations and listen to my chest for noises that show I might be retaining fluids in my lungs. I'm exhausted after they leave. It's hard to be up for visits and examinations when you're worn out from any effort at all.

"I wait for people who visit to come up with something to say other than, 'And how are you feeling today, George?' I want to reply, 'How the hell do you think I'm feeling? I have Lou Gehrig's disease, and I'm going to die soon. How would you feel?'

"Since I can't be left alone anymore, I wait for the home health aide to stay with me while you go to the university. And I wait for the sound of the garage door at the end of the day, because I know it's you getting home. I'm so happy to see you. I wait for you to fix my hot toddy and our dinner, and feed me. That pleases me.

"I wait for our nights out at the Old Brogue Pub to see my buddies and enjoy some Bushmills Irish whiskey. I love to tease you when you slide me in and out of the car using the green trash bag.

"I wait for you to take me upstairs to prepare me for bed. The evening ritual is exhausting for both of us as you undress me, seat me on the bidet, then dress me in my pajamas, you brush my teeth, get me into bed, rub and kiss my forehead, and tell me to stay put. That always makes me laugh. Sometimes I forget, and you have to scoop me up off the floor to put me back into bed, or call the neighbors for help. Finally, you had the gall to tell me that you ordered a hospital bed with side rails to keep me in bed when I forget. I don't like that, but you threaten me like Nurse Ratchet, 'You have your choice: either a hospital bed or the scuzziest nursing home I can find, and I've found two already.' So the dratted hospital bed arrives the next day.

"I'm always waiting for something to happen to me, or to be done to me. Time hangs on, and the loneliness creeps in. It haunts me.

"As I wait, I watch myself die a little every day. It's probably impossible for you to imagine the searing exhaustion I go through. Or to understand how frustrating and demeaning it is not to be able to do anything for myself. But you don't let me get away with whining. 'You can still breathe without any difficulty. So get off the pity pot!'

"At the end of the day, I wait for sleep, because that's the only time I feel better."

Sitting by George's bed the next morning when he awakened, I watched his eyes search the room until they landed on my face smiling at him. "Hey, there," I said, holding in my hand a ribbon attached to some jingle bells. "I'm going to tie these bells around your wrist. If you lose your whistle, you can shake your bells."

He laughed and said, "Phyllis, you are the craziest person I know and the dearest!"

I thought, *What a benefit to be crazy in this situation.*

Over breakfast, we talked about how we could help each other work through the monotonous, lonely moments.

"I know you miss going to your book club lunch because you can't feed yourself there. Two of your buddies called me recently and asked if we could have the book club lunch here. They miss your company and investment advice. I think it's a great idea. What do you think?"

Startled, George answered, "Can you handle that?" He grinned.

"I doubt it, but I can try, you crazy man. I'll put you on the phone today with Jim and you can discuss the details."

"That was nice of Jim to suggest this," George said.

I continued, "Next, since I need to learn as much as I can about investment strategies, you can teach me more about the principles of handling a portfolio. You've taught this many times at the university and your lecture notes aren't completely yellowed. Your brain is still alert. You can teach it again. I'll be your assistant and you can dictate your revised lecture notes to me. How does that sound?"

The old familiar, flyboy smile returned to his face, which seemed to bring color back to his cheeks. He said, "Have you been up all night planning this?"

"Of course," I answered.

And so we went on, waiting together.

LIFE'S SIMPLE PLEASURES

"I can't whistle any more."

One spring morning in 2002, I went upstairs to help George with our usual routine of getting him out of bed, to the bathroom, and downstairs for breakfast. He was strangely quiet, and I thought I saw tears sliding out of the corner of his eyes. I smiled at him and that often did the trick to make his face relax and smile back. He used to tell Dr. Hank, our hospice physician, "I go to sleep at night seeing Phyllis' smile, and I wake in the morning seeing her smile." He'd grin and say, "What a lucky man I am."

Not so this morning. He didn't smile back. "Do you want to rest a little longer?" I asked. He indicated yes, nodding his head.

"Okay, when you're ready to get up, just whistle, baby, and I'll be back," I said and turned to leave the room.

In a faint voice he answered, "I can't whistle any more."

An aching silence followed as I realized what he'd said. I spun around to look at him. I knew then the reason for the tears that were pooling on his eyelashes. He needed time to collect his dignity before he faced the day. George had lost another of the simple pleasures that he'd known since a child: his capacity to whistle.

I went over and hugged him and said, "We'll figure another way for you to call me. Why not rest a few minutes while I go down and fix breakfast. I'll be back."

He nodded assent.

While I was making coffee and old fashioned oatmeal for him, I thought of the stories he'd told me about when he was five years old and Stella, his mother, would say, "Selby, you're going to blow your teeth straight out of your mouth if you keep up that whistling. Stop it, and start being a gentleman." Stella would add, "I can't stop you from calling me Stella, but don't you ever forget that I'm your mother." George called her Stella until she died in her nineties. She called him Selby.

George told her he hated the name Selby. It was a sissy name. Selby was George's middle name and his mother's maiden name. George wanted to be called George, his first name and his father's middle name. Because he was embarrassed when Stella introduced him as Selby, he'd whistle to show his dislike of the name. He thought Selby was no name for a growing boy and a man.

George continued to whistle as he grew up. It

reminded him of Huck Finn and Tom Sawyer and other literary characters that he enjoyed reading as a child. He told me, "I used to climb a tree, take Huck, an apple and read all afternoon so Stella couldn't find me and tell me what to do."

Other times he said that whistling gave him a sense of peace that no one could take away from him because he went deep inside his own world when he whistled. It kept the bossiness and meanness out of what he saw all around him, especially as a fighter pilot in Korea and Vietnam. He also whistled because he was incredibly good at it.

Whistling was also a sentimental connection for us. When we met at my home on July 10, 1970 for our blind date, the first sound I heard from George was a whistle as he leapt up the stairs to my town house and saw me jump over Princess, my blind standard poodle.

It was a great start to a long friendship and life together.

When I was about to go upstairs to get George out of bed, I heard a strange noise from the third floor. When I walked to the bottom of the stairs to the third floor, I heard a painful sobbing. I raced up to the bedroom and found George slumped over his desk, his hands over his head on the glass top, tugging at pieces of his hair. He was sobbing convulsively and hyperventilating.

His tears were so heavy, his nose was dripping and his face had big red blotches everywhere. He couldn't talk.

I tried to comfort him, standing beside his chair, hugging him, and gently rocking him back and forth. I let him cry. It was the first time I'd seen my husband really cry in the more than thirty years I'd known him, yet he'd withstood so much pain, especially in his mid years when his wife unilaterally ended their marriage and his life with his children.

He howled like an unhappy toddler with his head-back and his mouth open. His eyes were weary and he slumped his shoulders again. "Who's going to take care of you when I go? I can't anymore. Promise me you'll move back to Boston where your cousins live. They'll take care of you."

"George, it's all right for you to cry. You need to do that. You've held back for too many years. We can talk about where I will live later." I was relieved to see him finally let go of the disappointments that he'd carried for so long.

While I wanted to cry and let go myself, I felt I had to be strong for him since he was dependent upon me to keep us going. I felt terrified for him and wanted to help him. But I was relieved in some ways because I felt there were many times since I'd known him when he had needed to cry and let go of his rage.

Yet, I had never seen him do so before today.

There had been other difficult losses with this disease, other ways in which George could no longer protect me or himself. Giving up his guns was terrible for him. Like many men, George had an emotional connection to objects. He enjoyed fine machinery: guns, airplanes, and cars. As an engineer he appreciated the precision of these tools, a precision that reflected his personality.

The most special of his three guns was one he carried in Korea that he had to use when he was shot down in his airplane. He'd learned to be an expert marksman as a teenager in the New Jersey National Guard. He prided himself on that accomplishment, but he never hunted or killed animals with his guns. Target practice was fun but that was all. When living alone before we were married, he'd been burglarized twice, but he was not home. He wanted me to learn to shoot to have protection when he was away.

I didn't like guns in the house. But he kept a loaded one in the bedroom, which didn't help me sleep with any comfort. When he became ill and we had to move, I said the guns had to go—and not to the new house.

"I have too much to do and worry about without keeping track of guns. You can't use them, and I won't use them. And we have inquisitive grandchildren who get into everything."

He called several gun stores and sold them. He didn't tell me when he did it, but when he didn't speak to me for two days, I knew how deep the wound was for him. I didn't know if selling his guns was worse than giving up driving. At least he still had me as his driver, but he didn't have a gun as protection.

But this loss seemed worse. By now, George's sobbing was only a muffled noise. He was spent. I asked if he wanted to lie down for a few minutes before going to breakfast. "Please, and sit down beside me while I rest." He added, "I can't whistle for you anymore."

While I read, he slept for over an hour. He looked haggard and beaten. When he awakened, I said, "Hey, how about a cup of coffee and breakfast? Or would you rather have a shower first? Anna is away, so you have to put up with me today."

"I'd rather have you anytime. Let's do it," he grinned.

Freshly showered, shaved, and dressed, he looked like his old self again. The storm had passed. It was the start of a new day, figuring out ways for him to call me when he needed me.

George had experienced many hits in his life, but he'd managed to fly on one wing before, even though it might have been a rough trip.

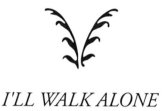

I'LL WALK ALONE

"Go have a good time with our friends. But don't pick up any men.
I'm not dead yet."

Several days after our fifteenth wedding anniversary in May 2002, I sat alone in the back row of a wooden,
A-framed Unitarian-Universalist church. The windowed
walls showed off the woods near the church, with newly
planted thickets of wild rose and shrubs, and fully developed hickory and birch trees. Growing up in New England, I always felt I was home in the presence of my favorite birch trees with their graceful, almost horizontal
branches. They guided me back to my foster homes as
I walked home from school, picking wild berries in the
woods.

The burning candles smelled like pine and
wildflowers. I was attending alone the wedding of two
friends because George was too tired to go—even in a
wheelchair. He told me, "Go have a good time with our
friends. But don't pick up any men. I'm not dead yet." I
asked one of his friends to stay while I was gone and help

him with his computer, as they both enjoyed jazz music.

Sitting alone in the back row, I didn't feel like I could stay for the entire service, even though George had company. The small church was full of family and close friends. Seeing the beauty and tenderness on the lovers' faces as they read their special written vows to each other, my heart flipped and my feet froze. But the informal service was short with only one musical piece. Like we did, our friends were entering into a second marriage later in life. They expected to live their remaining years without parental responsibilities, devoted to each other.

Automatically, I reached out to squeeze George's hand. Instead I felt the hardness of the wooden pew. My heart swelled with love as I thought of George's generosity of spirit. He insisted that I continue to live, while he was dying. "I want to be sure that our friends will be there for you after I'm gone," he said. He reminded me that our time was limited, but he wanted to feel confident I would be all right without him.

Like many people, I cry at weddings. I didn't feel conspicuous when I left with a wet face, after congratulating our friends. They hugged me and thanked me for sharing this special time with them. They knew the effort it was for me to leave George at home and come alone.

I had to give myself permission to walk away from my husband, go to work, and be company for my friends. I wanted to double up with the pain in my gut as I forced myself to leave him. But I knew that this was part of my responsibility to myself. Sometimes I questioned if I was being selfish, but I knew that soon I would be alone, and

I would need to live my life alone.

At times, I had to get outside the sickroom and participate in normal activities so ALS didn't suck away my identity. I knew I had to keep practicing so that when George died, I could still go on living. I couldn't forget how to live. But how do you do this when it means spending less time with the person you love?

Again, I grappled with the tension of opposites— —between being completely caring, and at the same time respecting my own need for space and healthy interactions with others. This was one of the hardest challenges I faced on this journey. It was so hard leaving George with someone else, especially when the nursing aide told me when I came home that he refused to eat his dinner until I returned. When I returned from teaching, I'd find him waiting for me wearing a big grin. "What's for dinner?" he'd say.

While I couldn't take away his loneliness, he eagerly awaited my stories about where I'd been and what I'd seen and heard. He was hungry to hear stories about my teaching. As a former professor, he often offered good suggestions on how to manage classroom issues.

We had a solid marriage—honest, caring, and open to compromise. It was gut wrenching to know we'd be losing this, but we didn't become ALS. However, there was still a big hole in my heart, even though I knew we were doing all we could to help each other. Oh, what mixed feelings I experienced.

I needed to survive: I wanted to go down the path of death with him. This tension itself was the intimacy that would bind us all our lives: how to connect yet not merge; how to respond yet not be absorbed; how to detach but not withdraw.

George often expressed his gratitude to me for the gift of spiritual security I gave him. He knew I'd watch out for him and he'd never be left alone. And we both knew that, however much he wanted to protect me, I would be alone.

HAPPY SECOND BIRTHDAY, GEORGE

"Phyllis, we're having so much fun, people outside are going to think we are doing something naughty."

It was now two years since my husband was told he had six months to live. The wicked disease was relentlessly devouring his body, eating its way through his arm and leg muscles, and making its way toward the diaphragm muscle he used to breathe. Just when his body adjusted to one change, without warning he dropped down to a lower plateau. George was too weary to have a big birthday party, but we still needed to celebrate his life, so we decided to celebrate with friends at a French restaurant in McLean, Virginia.

We met our friends, who were already waiting to help get George inside. He and I had made an agreement that we'd use the wheelchair only if someone wasn't there to meet us. Otherwise, we'd use the wheelchair to the door. I'd park it outside and get him seated inside. At that point, I'd put the wheelchair back in the car until we left.

Celebrating George's second ALS birthday, we

reminisced and carried on like normal folks. We were comfortable living our life in public, enjoying what was important to us: eating with friends and family.

We were all animated. I ordered champagne for all of us to celebrate this special evening. I always brought straws when we ate out because George could drink only with a straw. "I use a straw so I can drink faster than Phyllis, and she is fast," George teased. "She gets two drinks in before dinner." He winked at me.

We laughed with him and exchanged funny happenings since we were last together.

I noticed a young woman, to my left in the corner, watching us as she bent down to sip her drink. Slight in build, she had short blond hair, and a broad smile. Our eyes connected as if we were talking to one other. Her eyes shifted from mine to watch George. We were laughing so hard; I dropped some food in his lap. "Phyllis, you've had too much champagne," he joked. "You're cut off."

A few minutes later, the waiter brought more glasses of champagne. I said he must have the wrong table, but he told us these were complimentary. I glanced at the woman in the corner, and our smiles connected again. I raised my glass to her, as she nodded.

Later, I asked the waiter if the champagne was from the lady in the corner. He said yes. She had just flown into town to pick up her dress for her wedding the next day. Her parents owned the restaurant.

Apparently life was good for her at the moment and she wanted to share that. It's the best way to honor someone you love. She also must have admired the connection between George and me as I fed him and gave him his champagne and his pleasure with our group of partiers. She enjoyed watching us laughing and smiling under less than favorable conditions and she wanted to pass her joy in that on as well. When she stood to leave, she gave me a slight wave with her right hand and smiled. I smiled back knowing she was a soul-mate.

Later that evening, when I kissed my husband goodnight, he looked up at me and said, "Thank you for another great birthday party, Phyl. But don't put lilies on my chest tonight, dear. I'm still having fun."

About ten days later, it was time to vote in Virginia. George was a life-long Republican, but I loved him anyway, in spite of it. He had little to say about politics and resisted my efforts to change his mind. He would listen to me patiently as I ranted about George Bush's latest 'plans' and his leadership capabilities, or lack thereof.

After awhile he would say, "Phyllis, why are you surprised? You think all politicians are corrupt." He was right, but it didn't stop me from speaking up.

In the past, when we lived in Great Falls, I persuaded George to have election dinners at our roomy home every two years. He invited his Republican friends, and I invited my Democratic friends. We had two big television sets in different rooms so everyone could mingle around as they wanted. These parties were fun because my friends were academics who tended to be liberal and his friends were conservative military folks. What a mix of fireworks—just like the Fourth of July. But everyone came to our parties prepared for noise, arguing, and fun—plus good food and wine.

His friends often asked him, "George, how do you put up with Phyllis' independence and stubbornness? But she sure is a good cook."

George would laugh and say, "I just let the bird fly. She always comes home to me."

George's continued deterioration made me realize that the November 2002 election was the last one he'd participate in. However, there was one problem: he couldn't use his arms or fingers to work the voting apparatus. I'd need to push the buttons for him.

"George, do you want to vote next Tuesday?" I asked him. We voted at Westgate Elementary School, only a few blocks away. "I can call ahead and find out if it is possible for me to vote for you. Also, I need to find out what I should bring to verify who we are, since we don't have the same last names."

"I'd like to vote, Phyl, but how am I going to do that? I can barely work my computer keys. I can't even pinch you on the bottom."

"Oh, that's just because you haven't tried to pinch me recently, George. I know I'm not gorgeous, but I'm all you have, darling. I'll push the keys for you in the voting booth. I'll just explain to them that you have ALS and can't use your fingers." I added, "I can get a letter from Dr. Hank verifying this fact just like you had to get a letter from your parents when you needed special privileges at school."

With a smirk, he said, "We don't need a letter. I'm sure you're enough to scare them."

"Thanks, George, but we have to do this right to convince them. Since I work the elections, I know how sticky they are on details and any variation from the rules. You know that from being in the military too. We'll use the transport wheelchair in the back of the car to get you in and out."

So I dressed George to look like he was tired and ill. I combed his hair, but didn't part it. And I didn't let him look in the mirror. After putting his night wool cap on his head, I slipped on and tied his old, dirty tennis shoes. Brooks Brothers didn't make it to the election place this time.

When we arrived George put his head on his chest and scrunched down looking like he wanted to become invisible. It was a good thing that he was hard of hearing. I made sure that he was turned away from us so he couldn't hear me talk to the officials. If we were going to pull this off, he had to be quiet and look sick. I took along a big blanket to cover his legs.

I chose the best time to arrive, when there would be a long line so that the officials would need to move people along quickly. I put our credentials on the table: our marriage certificate, both of our driver's licenses, and a letter from hospice. Our request was quickly approved, and I wheeled George off to the booth and pulled the curtain.

When we were safely inside, I took George's hat off

because it was warm in there. We looked at the machine, and George gave me instructions on how to use it.

"Get off it, George. What's the Hell's the matter with you? I help people with these machines all the time. Now, I have a big surprise for you, George. You're about to become a Democrat. I'm so tired of you canceling my votes all these years."

He stared at me with horror on his face. He was used to my pranks, but he couldn't comprehend I'd do this in the voting booth. Finally, when I grinned at him, we both started to laugh uproariously.

"Isn't this wonderful, George? It's your last chance on this earth to correct all your sins of the past. As a Democrat, you are now converted and saved. The good God in the sky will let you in to sit beside him because of this conversion."

We continued to laugh heartily until tears slid down our cheeks. There wasn't much for us to laugh about anymore. We needed every little bit of cheer we could get.

"Phyllis, since we're having so much fun, people outside are going to think we are doing something naughty in here."

We continued laughing. "But I think we better start voting. Do you know whom you're voting for? Do you want to see my list?"

I pressed the keys he wanted as he monitored my selections. I told him he was a lost soul. After pulling the curtain open, I turned him around in the wheelchair to find many people looking at us, wide-eyed. No one was laughing like we were. I whisked him away in his wheel-chair, his head on his chest, the way he entered earlier.

Later, he enjoyed telling this story to his friends with relish and considerable embellishment. He had had a good time at the polls.

But you have to admire him. He was a real Republican. He got out to vote.

III

NOVEMBER 2002—MARCH 2003

CARING FOR GRANDPA GEORGE

"Careful, woman, you're maiming my manhood."

We usually shared Thanksgiving with our daughter and her family in Nashville, Tennessee, where they lived, or visited historic places together. But in 2002, George was too tired to travel any long distance so the family came to Virginia. Elated about their visit, George ordered new harmonicas and washboards for our granddaughters Claire and Lorna, who were seven and three-and-a-half years old. He was a looming figure in their lives.

They shared a lively interest in both making music and making noise. George and Claire started jamming together on the harmonica and wooden washboard before she was four. During this visit, he wanted to give them new harmonicas and steel washboards—a replica of the real wooden washboards used by women to wash clothes before modern machines. I remember as a child during the Great Depression living in foster homes how, with a bar of hand-made lye soap, we scrubbed and rubbed the dirty laundry against the ridges on the wooden washboards placed in washtubs. Our skinned knuckles were red and sore for days. Then it was time to start again.

George had learned to play the washboard when he was stationed in Nashville for Army boot camp in 1943. Early in the 20th century, jug bands used the washboard as a percussion instrument for Zydeco and jazz. The ridges on the boards were made with metal surfaces then which gave more sound. The players used a variety of items like spoons and thimbles to tap the metal ridges. It was considered a 'poor man's' instrument created for musicians who lacked the money to purchase real instruments.

As usual, in mid-afternoon when the family arrived, there was exuberant hollering as everyone hugged, ran around the car grabbing bags of stuff they brought, dropped things in the driveway, and squealed like piglets happy to be together again. When we were settled in the family room, George gave the girls the washboards and new harmonicas. Everyone was thrilled except, perhaps, the parents, who blinked their eyes at the sight of yet more noisemakers.

During our past visits, the girls and George jammed like other musicians. They sat on the floor in the family room with their instruments, singing and playing. There was no prepared music, just the free flowing noise they were able to squeeze out of their harmonicas and whip up on the washboards. George named them the Ramage Ragtime Band.

He loved ragtime and jazz from his earliest childhood memories when his father played violin in the New Jersey Symphony Orchestra. His father also played jazz violin and George had a thirst for this kind of music all his life. His piano teacher and his mother insisted he play Edward MacDowell's "To a Wild Rose," a haunting classical piano solo that ladies, like his mother, having tea would appreciate. He refused to continue his lessons.

To add to their musical adventure, I bought the girls an oversized six-foot piano mat that we stretched out in front of the real piano. They jumped on it immediately, stomping back and forth on the keys that gave off realistic instrumental sounds. But the mat had more than piano music: it had eight different built-in instruments such as drums, guitar, banjo, trumpet and others.

What a whooping party we had when the girls and I jumped on the mat together—what musical rapture. We chuckled as we sang made-up songs, and pushed each other off the mat. Bouncing spontaneously in the air from key to key, I felt like a little girl again, deliriously free from the sorrows of our journey.

The next day was Thanksgiving. We were having dinner at our favorite country inn, 1763 Inn, in Upperville, Virginia. At this point, George had to be pushed up the side ramp by wheelchair because the stairs into the restaurant were steep and narrow.

I parked in a temporary spot near the front door and put George in the travel wheelchair before I went inside to find Uta, the proprietor. She followed me outside to the car and whisked George away up the side ramp into the restaurant. Claire walked at his side, holding onto his hand. George didn't know what hit him but he was grinning like he won the lottery.

By the time I parked the car, and the rest of us climbed the stairs to the dining room, Uta had placed George at the head of the table. The wheelchair was nowhere to be seen. Claire, sitting beside her grandfather, was beaming at their accomplishment.

"Grandpa said I could help him eat," Claire announced from her position of authority.

George winked at me and invited us to join him for dinner. Part of our usual ritual was for Lorna to put paper covered straws at each place so we all drank with the same type of straws as Grandpa George.

Whenever we visited the inn, Uta and George were old sparring buddies, always teasing, sharing ideas on the stock market, her latest trips, and tennis. She was a real pro, tall, strong and determined. Even though the rest of us ate Thanksgiving dinner, Uta surprised George with his favorites: Bushmills, sauerbraten, knockwurst, red cabbage, coleslaw, apple strudel, and German Forest cake.

George said that the beef was tender, and the red cabbage had a nice bite to it. We sniffed the vinegary, clove aromas from the sauerbraten and the many spices from the familiar steaming apples. He was beaming. Tenderness came from every direction toward him, and I felt the privilege of not being alone to love and care for our Gentleman George.

After a long dinner telling funny stories and looking out the windowed walls at the pond, at the familiar swan guarding her family of three tennis balls, the same three ducks quacking as if they were daft, the spraying waterfalls, and luscious green hills, we prepared to leave. Claire helped Grandpa George walk from the table to the outside ramp where the wheelchair was parked. Uta saw them and sprinted to the door, with Lorna close behind. As Uta wheeled the chair down the ramp, Claire and Lorna tucked their little fingers in each of his useless hands.

George was finally happy in his wheelchair because he felt so comfortable and accepted. I saw peace on his glowing face. Tears of joy bubbled up inside me as I watched the compassion and empathy our young children shared with their grandpa. My heart ached because I knew that this was the last time they'd see Grandpa George. We wouldn't be able to travel for our usual Christmas holiday together at the Homestead, a mountain resort in Virginia.

When I saw the depth of love shared between the girls and George, I felt cheated for them by this cruel disease. But they were unaware of my thinking and were busy building their own memories and relationships with their grandpa. Years later when they looked at family albums, they would remember. The bundle of memories that crosses generations are lost if we enjoy only living and hide the dying from children.

The truth about sickness can't be kept from kids. Children need adequate information to help them understand and cope with what they are experiencing. They perceive dying and death differently at varying developmental levels, but they always perceive them. As they listen to adults talk, they absorb all they can, and discard the rest. They will know how to find their way in when they're curious and eager to participate. Such was the case with our grandchildren.

When we got home in the early evening, we jammed for another hour, while the parents left for a walk. As an engineer, George applied his skills to solve many problems resulting from this destructive disease. That evening he came up with an idea of how he could hold his harmonica with his constantly declining arms. I taped a podium onto the table where George sat, and he fixed his elbows on the table, elevating his arms to hold the harmonica by bending his face towards the podium. I put the other harmonicas and washboards on the table so everyone could switch instruments if they wanted to.

Even using all his strength, the effect from trying to hold the harmonica reduced George's breathing capacity. Although he didn't make much sound, he was happy to be playing again. Claire made lots of noise on the washboard. Lorna and I ran up and down on the piano mat. We made strange sounds because we jumped from instrument to instrument so fast. Claire, seeing George's difficulty, went over and said, "Grandpa, let me try your big harmonica, and you can try this new washboard."

I put some thimbles on his fingers so he could move them back and forth across the board that Claire laid on the table in front of him. His eyes lit up and widened when the jazz sounds burst from his washboard. To take the focus off him, I rejoined Lorna as we backed them up, jamming on the piano mat. I also didn't want anyone to see me cry at the tender caring that Claire gave her grandpa.

After Claire switched to playing the real piano, George said, "Claire, that sounds like good jazz you're playing."

Little Lorna answered earnestly, "That's not good jazz, Grandpa George. That sucks." Her honesty broke us up and we all doubled over laughing. Lorna looked at us bewildered about what she'd said that caused so much laughter. By then, George was exhausted, so I took him upstairs to get ready for bed.

That night, George slept eleven hours without getting up to go to the bathroom. A few weeks earlier, I'd asked hospice to find George a hospital bed with side rails. He'd been falling out of his twin bed during the night, or forgetting to call me when he needed me. When we moved into the townhouse, I'd bought twin beds so I could get some sleep. Sometimes I didn't hear him get up, and he wouldn't ring his call device. I hoped the side rails would remind him to call me instead of getting up alone.

Two weeks earlier, Lynn, our physical therapist, also suggested a hospital bed because the increased height would reduce the back strain for me. She'd watched me when I bent down to get George out of the low twin bed and was concerned that I would injure myself again. A month earlier, I'd torn a meniscus in my left knee moving George from the wheelchair to the bidet. I still got cortisone shots in the knee to handle the pain and swelling, plus I had to wear a leg brace.

George was not happy when the hospital bed arrived with the Geo-Matt polyurethane foam mattress topper that I'd requested. We used these toppers in the hospital because the unique design of the individual foam cells was sized to fit each area of the body. It helped to prevent pressure ulcers for those patients who couldn't move themselves. George was quickly moving in that direction.

He insisted that the twin bed remain in our bedroom in case he wanted to use it. I told him how difficult it was for me to get him out of the twin bed, and we certainly didn't need three beds in the bedroom. The twin bed would go to another room. We could bring it back if the hospital bed didn't work out. He scowled at me, but stopped when I reached over and hugged him.

"You've told me many times you want to be sitting up and conscious when you die. This bed will make it easier for you because I can raise the head with a tap of this electric button." Then I added, "And if you don't stay in bed at night, I can make you into a sandwich with these buttons."

His eyes widened in horror, but when he saw me grinning he said, "OK, I get it. You make the rules, right?"

"Yes, sir." I said. But, in truth, being in charge of a vulnerable, grown man you love beyond all reason was gut wrenching.

After his big day Thanksgiving, George was still sleeping the next morning when I went down to make his breakfast. When I came back to wake him, I saw the back ends of two little girls racing into our bedroom. They scampered up onto his hospital bed, asking permission after they landed. I ran to the bed in time to see George's eyes fly open. The force of their landing wasn't soft, and it must have hurt him.

"Grandpa George! Come to breakfast," they shouted in chorus.

"OK, but where's grandma?" he asked.

"Here I am," I said. "You girls go downstairs while I get Grandpa up. Daddy is making waffles. You save some for us, okay?"

And away they went as fast as they arrived.

I looked at George and expected to hear him groaning from such an abrupt awakening. But his face was radiant. His darlings were still here.

After a busy morning of activity and lunch, I suggested that the family do something together like a movie so Grandpa George could take a nap. George had to economize his strength because it wasn't renewable. After one day of effort like Thanksgiving, he needed at least a day, or even two, to recuperate.

The girls took Grandpa upstairs for his nap, and crawled in his bed to tell him stories before he went to sleep. By the time I arrived in the bedroom, they were all napping in the bed. They looked like a row of puppies lying on their backs with their hands up as though they were waiting to have their bellies rubbed. I wished I had a camera.

George never tired of the girls caring for him. His greatest joy was to be cared for by family members because he was so comfortable with them. To George, few pleasures exceeded the sweet smells and hugs of his grandchildren and the ordinary moments they shared as they fed him, washed his face, combed his hair, and told Grandpa George he couldn't go out and play unless he ate all his lunch.

Later in the afternoon when everyone was awake, I gave the girls another gift that I thought would be fun, but quieter than jamming: the Classic Jumbo Builder set of tinker toys. The box was tall, and cylindrical in shape and it made lots of noise when the delighted girls shook it several times. Making noise was their passion. Invented early in the 20th century, these were the tools of American tinkerers. They've been classic toys for children for generations.

Using their imaginations, either working as a team or separately, the girls connected the simple wooden rods and spools, shaped and sorted by size, color, and type to build varying structures. George lay still in his bed, quietly taking in the action. Excited, the girls climbed onto his bed and emptied the boxes in his lap.

"Grandpa, you could walk down the hall if you had a walker. I'm going to make you one," Claire said. She busied herself sorting out her long pieces and the shorter ones. "Did you get this ALS thing flying through the air when you were flying in those wars?" she asked nonchalantly.

"No one knows, Claire, but I think that's as good an explanation as any I've heard so far."

When Grandpa told Claire he couldn't hold on to

a walker, she said she would build him crutches to put under his arms. When she'd finished her work, she told Grandpa she was ready for him to get up to try his new crutches.

I looked at George, and he looked at me as we tried to figure out how to manage this arrangement. I got him out of bed, and the girls put wobbly crutches they'd made for him with tiny pieces of wooden tinker toys under his arms. Then each held a hand to form a parade to the elevator. I grabbed George firmly by the back of his sweat pants to support him on his trip to the elevator.

"Careful, woman, you're maiming my manhood," he joked.

George clenched his teeth and sucked in his breath to concentrate on standing tall.

So Claire and Lorna had given one more message of love to Grandpa George during their visit—crutches made from tinker toys.

Claire continued to watch her grandpa every minute. I knew I could relax and let her enjoy her position. She took care of several tasks—feeding him, guiding him around the house using the elevator—my new caring assistant. We certainly don't need to be medically credentialed to help a loved one during the final days.

Our grandchildren were thrilled because they had done something to help and care for their grandpa, whom they loved very much. I put a smile on my face when I saw him so I wouldn't cry from seeing so much love from these children. He was ecstatic, his face radiant.

At such a time in one's life—and impending

death—the importance of family is central. The beauty of these children working so earnestly to care for their grandpa, who wore a slaphappy grin on his face during their entire visit, pushed me into simultaneous joy and sorrow.

PEOPLE WHO NEED PEOPLE

"Get the wheelchair in the car, and let's go!"

The holidays were nearing an end. George's strength was declining so much that he decided he wasn't strong enough to attend the usual New Year's Eve West Point class party. It was a tough decision for him. He said, "I don't want to let my friends down, but I think I'm too tired to be much fun."

"All right. I know your friends will understand. I'll give them a call and explain." I added, "I told you last week that our neighbors, Susan and Larry, invited us to their neighborhood party. If you want to go for a short time, I need to call them. We can leave the party anytime."

"Let's do that. You'd enjoy it," he answered.

"Yes, I won't have to drive. After I call them, I'm going to run to the store. I'm supposed to take a salad. Are you comfortable where you are? I don't want you getting into mischief while I'm gone. Will you promise to stay in that chair?"

"I want to go to the bathroom first. Will you make

your special fresh fruit salad?"

"Yes, I will. Now let's get you sorted out so I can shop."

The next evening we went to our friends' party, walking the short distance across the town-house street. I decided to leave the food at home until I had him comfortable upstairs in our neighbors' house. They didn't have an elevator so I knew I would need to help him climb the stairs to the second level.

When I rang the bell, our host, Larry, opened the door immediately and offered to guide George up the stairs to the party. I told him I was going home to collect the salad, wine and Bushmills.

When I returned to the party, George was holding court in a leather high-back Queen Anne chair, smiling and already drinking Bushmills with a long straw from his glass on the table next to him. I took the salad, wine and other items into the kitchen to Susan, the hostess. The musky smell of fresh baked bread and lasagna cooking in the oven tickled my nostrils.

I was overwhelmed as I hugged Susan and Larry and thanked them. What a tender, sensitive and gracious gesture to remember that George liked Bushmills, and that he couldn't hold his own drink. By putting it on a table next to him with a long straw, he could bend down and enjoy it. Such is the beauty of the friendship that lit our way, making the quality of our life a richer and more loving experience.

We were the last of the dozen or so guests to arrive. Most were middle-aged couples who enjoyed discussing business and finance issues. Several like George were retired military and reserve officers, so they had great stories to share.

Sipping wine, I sat back and watched George, engaged and animated the entire evening. Even while I was feeding him fruit salad, lasagna, flank steak, fresh bread, and chocolate cake, he still participated one-hundred percent.

The evening was a happy one for everyone.

When the evening was over, Larry held George's arm and helped him walk across the street and into our elevator. His legs were wobbly, but he didn't stumble. As I watched the two men, I felt a rock in the bottom of my stomach because I knew this would be his last New Year's Eve Party. But George was a happy man starting out his first day of 2003.

When I tucked him into bed that night, he whispered to me again, "Don't put lilies on my chest tonight, dear. I'm still having fun."

He slept for fourteen hours without calling to go to the bathroom, or trying to crawl over the side rails of the hospital bed.

George's frailty continued to show more every day, as we descended from one plateau to the next one. As his body continued to break down, George settled into a new rhythm of living. Then the rhythm changed again. The time between plateaus was decreasing. That is the nature of ALS. You hang onto each plateau as long as you can.

I made sure George took a nap each afternoon, so when he met his friends for dinner, he sometimes had enough energy to feed himself. This pleased him, and he finally got over the idea that to nap in the daytime was a sign of laziness. He still wanted to go out once or twice a week to see his friends for dinner at the pub, and I invited friends in for dinner at least once a week.

While he could still travel safely and I could manage to get him in and out of the car, I decided I'd better get him in for a haircut. George would only go to a real, old-fashioned, manly barbershop, not some hair salon. I called our neighbor, Ken, who owned a barbershop in McLean and asked if I could bring George in his wheelchair. Ken already knew he was ill. I asked him to give George the 'works,' whatever that was, because I didn't know what to ask for.

Later that month, I told George he was going for a morning treatment at the barbershop. He was so excited, he said, "Get the wheelchair in the car, and let's go!"

When we arrived, I rolled George into the barbershop. Ken was there and immediately pushed George close to the barber chair. Another man helped Ken lift George up and into the barber chair. By this time, he had lost over fifty pounds, which made him easier to lift. George sank back into the leather chair.

Grinning like a Cheshire cat, I slid away to the corner where I hid so I wouldn't disturb the men's chatter and laughter. The jokes, stories, and teasing were delicious as the men shared their maleness. I wanted George to enjoy every minute of what I knew would be his last haircut.

He told them about his father taking him to the barbershop as a child. He'd listen and absorb the smells of tobacco, musky odors, and shaving cream as he watched his father getting his haircut and massage. He said this was the only place his father smoked his pipe. It smelled like clove and cherries, and was their secret.

I watched and listened from my inconspicuous corner. George always appreciated the art of manliness: horses, guns, and leather. When I dressed him in his flying jacket, he'd say, "Leather only smells and gets better with time." Before he lost the use of his hands, he'd polish his shoes with Kiwi black shoe polish. I can still smell that heavy tar. It made me sick and I refused to do it after he became incapacitated.

But the smell of shaving cream in the shop caught my attention. As Ken shaved him with a straight-edge razor, which George used to do himself, George's face was lit up and jolly. For nearly two years, he had had to accept me shaving him with an electric razor, not a manly way to shave. But because of my arthritic hands, I wasn't about to take on a straight-edge razor.

After watching George get a facial and neck massage, then get tipped back in the chair to enjoy a relaxing shampoo and cooling conditioner followed by a hot soothing towel, I decided to read my book. He was clearly in orbit. I understood then how important it was for him to be with his male friends in a male environment. It was fun, simple, safe, and accepting regardless of what you looked like or felt like. And more than that, our friend Ken gave all this service to George as a gift.

A few weeks later, we agreed to meet friends at the Old Brogue Pub. What had been a snowstorm turned into a blizzard as I drove. Traffic was crawling at five to ten miles per hour. Cars were sliding, but no accidents so far. Since I had four-wheel drive, my SUV clung to the road. I debated turning around but we were almost at the pub. When I asked George what he wanted me to do, he said, "Phyl, our friends will be expecting us." Sometimes I wondered if he thought I was Wonder Woman, or if he was just plain crazy.

When we finally arrived, the pub owner, Mike Kearney, and our friend, Harvey, were outside shoveling a parking place for us. In minutes, they had the wheelchair out of my trunk and had whisked George away into the pub. It was the first time that George ever went into a restaurant in his wheelchair. It happened so fast that he didn't realize what happened.

As I watched these men move so quickly to protect their friend and get him inside to the warmth of friends, good food, and drink, I understood, at least a little, the significance of maleness and the pub. It's a safe place for men to get together, face a lousy day, and be distracted from their troubles. This was what George really needed after a day of being with women caregivers and his wife, or just being alone.

We ate, and he drank his Bushmills, listening to one of the servers play hearty Irish music on his guitar. When the evening was over, our friends Harvey and Dianne followed us home to help me get George out of the car. That evening I had struggled to get him into the car, and I knew I wouldn't be able to safely get him out. The old trick of sliding him with the plastic trash bag wasn't adequate any more. I knew it was the last time I could move him into the car by myself.

Our evening reminded me again of how simple are the real pleasures of living—being with friends in the pub, sharing the joys of friendship, and caring for each other.

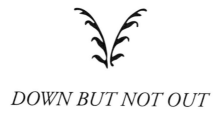

DOWN BUT NOT OUT

"I was on my way, but I forgot something."

After dinner in early February 2003 I helped George
into our private elevator to ride to the third floor to get
ready for bed. After I closed the elevator doors and turned
to smile at him, he looked at me with a fixed stare.

"Are you okay?" I asked.

"Yes, but I'm really tired."

As I moved around to be ready to open the elevator
doors, I felt George falling against me, fast. My knees
crumbled as his dead weight pushed us both to the floor.
Knowing the timer gave us only three seconds to open
the elevator before the lights turned off, I rolled out from
under him, placing his head on the floor. Grabbing the
inside accordion metal elevator door and shoving it back
to the wall, I was able to pull down the handle to open the
outside door.

Turning back, I looked at George's chalk-white
face. Leaning down to his face to feel for air coming from
his nose or mouth, I lay my fingers on his wrist for a pulse,

while calling his name. When he didn't answer, I slapped his face. He still didn't react, and his rapid, thin pulse was barely perceptible.

I ran into the bedroom, grabbed a blanket to cover him, and a pillow to put under his head, which I cuddled in my lap. I rubbed his face, especially his forehead, which he particularly liked. I talked to him about our friends coming for dinner the next night to watch *Casablanca*, one of our old-time favorites.

I felt the tension pulling on me to start doing CPR to get him breathing again. As a nurse, I wanted to resuscitate him by compressing his chest, an important first step in CPR. Instead, as his wife, I talked with him about this. Even though he didn't answer me, I felt he heard me.

"George, you look so peaceful and you're home. I'm keeping my promise to you. I won't resuscitate you."

When he didn't respond for several more minutes, I pulled down the elevator phone, stepped into the hallway, and dialed the hospice nurse on call and explained the situation.

"Have you called 911?" She asked.

"No, and I don't intend to."

"Why not?"

My heart did something funny in my chest. "We've been in your program for over ten months because my husband wants a peaceful death at home. He signed a medical directive to have no 911, no CPR, no resuscitation, and no life-saving devices."

This conversation brought home to me again

how important it is for everyone to be able to make their own end of life decisions and for these to be carried out, whether or not doctors or other health professionals agree with the patient's wishes.

The line was silent. About to hang up, I added, "I promised my husband he would die peacefully at home with no trips to the emergency room. As his trustee, I will respect his wishes and signed directives."

The silence on the line was palpable.

Finally, I said, "By the way, if my husband doesn't regain consciousness, you have to come here to pronounce him dead. I need to get back to my husband." I felt dizzy with the tension.

She agreed to come. I called my friends Dianne and Harvey to come help me get him out of the elevator.

Returning to George on the elevator floor, I found him curled on his left side, barely moving as he tried to turn over. I kneeled down beside him. "George, can you hear me? This is Phyllis. Are you okay?"

I touched his right wrist to feel for his pulse. It was faint but steady.

He stopped moving and didn't answer for a couple of minutes.

"Do you want me to help you?" I asked.

Suddenly his eyes opened. He looked at me with glazed eyes and no sign of recognition.

"Where am I?"

"George, this is Phyllis. You're home. Can you hear me?"

He answered, "I was on my way, but I forgot

something."

Thrilled to hear his voice, I hugged him and worked to make him comfortable for a moment by rubbing and kissing his forehead as I did every night when I settled him in bed. I thought I saw a flicker of recognition in his eyes.

"You just said you forgot something. You forgot me," I said.

"Oh, Phyllis, you're so silly. Nobody could forget you," he said, as his old, devilish grin crept up the sides of his face.

At that moment, I felt like smacking him, and probably would have if I hadn't been so happy. The stubborn ole mule rider was doing his thing again.

"Where were you?" I asked.

Glowing, George said, "On a trip. It was fun."

"I'm glad you had a good time. You scared the hell out of me."

"Sorry. Do I have to stay on the floor forever?" he asked.

"No, but since you're warm and comfortable, I'm not going to lift you by myself. Harvey and Dianne should be here any moment. Why not enjoy our funny family pictures on these walls. I put them there for you to enjoy when you ride the elevator."

He laughed. "Okay, sit here with me, please."

Our friends arrived shortly thereafter and helped me move him into the bathroom, where he was seated on his 'Bidet' throne when the nurse arrived.

George was holding court like a king on his throne

in the bathroom. "When he's finished," she asked, "please take him to his bed so I can talk with him." To which George answered, "I may be a while."

I offered her a cool drink or tea and gave her a comfortable chair to sit in. Then I returned to George to get him moving. He was in no hurry.

Eventually, I got him back to bed and the young nurse asked, "What happened?"

"I tried to pat Phyllis on the fanny in the elevator, but I missed and fell," he said.

His irreverent spirit didn't go over well with our young nurse. She said nothing as she continued to examine him, checking his blood pressure, pulse, and respirations, all of which had returned to normal. Since he fell on me, he had no physical injuries. The nurse left without asking any further questions, or leaving us any instructions.

No one even asked about me.

Several days later when George, a great storyteller, was joking about this story with some of our friends, several were indignant and shocked, showing their disdain of me by saying, "That's terrible, Phyllis. You should have called 911. He could have died in the elevator."

I wanted to say to them, "So what if he'd died? Why should I drag him to an emergency room to die when he made me promise him that he would die peacefully at home with no resuscitation?" But I said nothing. They wouldn't understand.

Finally, I asked George to stop sharing this story with our friends because I was tired of the criticism from people who knew I was a nurse. They failed to understand why I didn't act to save my husband from dying, which most people feel is the worst possible outcome for anyone. Dying peacefully at home is still not an accepted choice. Instead, people focus on technical medicine available in modern hospitals in emergency rooms where doctors work like salesmen. Death remains the worst enemy for many people.

For us, George's victory would be that he was conscious when he died peacefully at home, relieved from the pain and suffering of ALS, but triumphant in the way he lived with it.

The next day at breakfast, George asked me to take over managing his investment portfolio. This was his last vestige of independence. We had turned another corner. It was his message to me that he was near the end and couldn't fight any more, not even to exist.

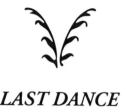

LAST DANCE

"May I have this dance for the rest of our life?"

When George and I met in July, 1970, I was thirty-seven and he was forty-six. We had lived through World War II, the Korean War and Vietnam. During those wars, hundreds of soldiers, sailors, and flyboys sporting snappy uniforms and dozens of well-coiffed Junior Hostesses packed USO (United Services Organizations) dance halls on Saturday nights.

During the Korean War, my nursing friends and I served as Junior Hostesses in Los Angeles at the USO dances and parties. We loved to kick off our clunky nurses' shoes and heavy, white, starched uniforms to slide into high-heels, lipstick and pretty dresses and ride the trolley car from the nurses' residence to the dance halls. We needed a break from our daily work at the hospital caring for sick and dying patients.

That night in July 1970, George and I reminisced about the stale smells of cigarette smoke—everyone smoked—beer, whiskey, and the forever burning coffee in the dance halls. For the hostesses, they served Coca-Cola in glass bottles since many of us weren't old enough to drink alcohol. We treasured the cozy, familiar touch of our dance partners' strong hands around our waists, pulling us close, but not so close that the senior hostesses would remind the men to behave respectfully. Graceful dancing was considered a "gracious way of living."

The sensuality of the opposite sex was pleasurable for everyone. During times of immense stress and confusion in the world, it was romantic and comforting to be part of a strong, supportive group, and to hold onto that strength as we danced the slow dances of waltz and fox trot. These dance halls, decorated in red, white, and blue crepe paper ribbons were home on the weekends for many estranged people away from home, and for those who wanted to give them comfort. Servicemen and hostesses happily forgot the war for a little while as they moved to the music.

It was the era of the big bands that brought our feet alive as we jumped to the call over the microphone, "Come on guys and gals, let's dance." While we often danced the fox trot and waltz, we all had the energy to break out and dance the 'swing', commonly known as jitterbugging. It was fast, and enlivened the room as the men either twirled us around until we were dizzy, tossed us into thin air, or slid us through their legs to the music of Glenn Miller playing *In the Mood* and Tommy Dorsey playing *Good Night, Sweetheart.*

As a serviceman, George attended these dances in WW II, when he was an aviation cadet in the Army, and during the Korean War, when he was a fighter pilot in the

Air Force.

As our blind date came to an end that warm July night in 1970, George and I were still talking about our hobbies and the activities we enjoyed. His interests were tennis, first, and golf, second. My interests were dancing, first, second, and third.

"I'd rather dance than eat," I told him.

"Really," he said. "I can't say I'd rather do anything more than eat, but well, maybe, fly. But I have to eat when I fly. The crew always serves me first. They know what a mean son-of-a-bitch I am when I'm hungry."

Over the years, our major social activities with our friends were tennis and dancing. I took tennis lessons, and George finally consented to attend dancing classes as long as I participated. As a junior high student in the 1930s, George had taken dancing classes. His mother made him attend Miss Molly's dance class in South Orange, New Jersey, because there weren't enough boys. George hated it. To him, it was sissy stuff, and he wanted no part of it. He'd rather be playing polo, or mucking stalls at the National Guard Horse Barn. He said he pretended to be sick. But his mother, a nurse, had figured out his scheme.

Saturday night became dance night for us with many of our friends. When George became ill, it was harder for him to keep his balance because his legs would buckle without warning. His weakened arms hung uselessly at his sides. But even though he couldn't hold a partner, that didn't stop our friends—or George—when they danced. The women threw their arms around his neck to hold him while they swayed to the music. His face radiated supreme joy as he moved his body on the dance floor.

I told him he had more rhythm now because he was using his body differently. I worried about him falling. But it never happened when he danced.

Now George was no longer capable of social dancing—nor social chitchat. In order to live entirely in the moment, expecting nothing in return, you had to be open to new dances together.

On our Saturday night dates, we had a new dance and a new dance hall: bidet dancing in our spacious master bathroom painted the soft daffodil yellow that George selected for this room and our master bedroom. It was a soft color embellished by the candles I always burned. I dimmed the lights and made it warm and welcoming like a dance floor. George often asked, "Why do you have candles burning everywhere?"

"Why not?" I answered. "Their fragrance is soothing to me and peaceful. Where's your romantic spirit?"

However, the bathroom didn't look, or smell like any dance hall that we remembered. It smelled like air freshener, the sweet smells of shit, Ivory soap—his favorite, Listerine mouthwash, toothpaste, and shaving cream. Occasionally, there was a whiskey smell from his hot toddy and a buttery or fig scent from my favorite oak-aged chardonnay that I kept in the bathroom for 'bidet' viewers and conversation. But our dance hall was good enough for us.

After I lifted him from the wheelchair, we shuffled along as I dragged his fragile body, and rocked back and forth to the music. I was still wearing a long, soft-hinged knee brace from an earlier knee injury.

We were a funny-looking sight. But he trusted me not to drop him. He would say, "I don't care what you do to me, but don't step on my toes."

I hugged him and said, "Don't you step on mine, either." The intimacy of dancing held us together. I reminded him of the song Judy Garland used to sing in the 1940's, "It only happens when I dance with you. . . ."

When I saw the love in his face as we slid across our tile dance floor, I was close to dissolving. I held him under his arms as we danced the two-step, probably the first dance we'd learned. His sapphire blue eyes showed deep love for our life together. We were lost in the love of the moment, lost in each other's faces, alone in our place in the world. Our bidet dance locked in the love we felt for each other, like the glue that sexual intercourse generates between lovers.

On Saturday night, March 15, 2003, George said, "May I have this dance for the rest of our life?" He never lost the graciousness that always marked him. I wondered at what point he knew he would die soon. When he asked me to dance, I felt he was giving me a subtle message, because he'd never asked me before. The joke with us was that I always asked him to dance.

I changed the selection to *Stardust* by Glenn Miller on the CD player. That song was part of our independent memories of the 1940s and WWII for George as a GI.

When the orchestra played *Stardust* at any dance, it was the signal that the dance was over.

As we glided slowly across the floor, we both knew our dancing together was almost over. This was our dance of life and death. You dance with the guy you bring to the party. You have to be willing to play new games, dance new dances together. We were as relaxed as an old couple could be. We were gentle with each other as we swayed to the music of Glenn Miller's *Stardust*, and sometimes we swayed too much because of my wounded knee. If anyone saw us they would know we were certifiably crazy.

"You are certainly the silliest person I have ever met, but also the dearest. Thank you," he said as he tried to pat me on my fanny.

After I had him settled into bed that last Saturday night, I poured myself a big glass of chardonnay and sank into my Jacuzzi tub for a long soak and meditation. Our dance that night felt different. His body temperature was cooler; the color on the sides of his face was grayer. I hadn't shaved him that morning at his request, and his whiskers stood out brisk and white. I wondered how his tired, decaying body could still push out more whiskers.

I felt that he had given me a message. This was our last dance. I was simultaneously plunged into distress and happiness. He would soon be free of this disease ravaging his body, but he would be gone from me, too, and I would have to live without him.

When the extension phone rang on my Jacuzzi tub, jolting me out of my reverie, I almost dropped it in the tub.

I remembered we had friends coming for lunch the next day. I debated if I should call them in the morning and cancel. Instead, I got out of the tub, went to the kitchen and made George's favorite dessert, key lime pie.

LAST MEAL, LAST BREATH

"Am I home?"

Monday, two days later, George was more tired and quiet than usual. I considered changing my schedule. After talking with him about how he felt, he said he would nap while I was gone. When I returned in the late afternoon, he had refused the dinner I prepared for the nursing assistant to feed him. He told her he'd like to eat with his wife. His nap had rejuvenated him.

He teased me, "Can't a guy get a good meal in this prison? I want steak for dinner." George was a steak and potatoes gourmet, but hadn't asked for either of these for months.

I was shocked. When I left for an appointment, he was barely able to talk, and now he wanted a steak dinner. *What was going on?*

As his nurse, I knew he shouldn't have steak. His digestive system was nearly inactive, and red meat is often the first food to be rejected by the dying. If he ate it, I knew he would be uncomfortable by that evening. But as his wife, I couldn't refuse him. He asked so little from me. I suspected he was giving me a subtle message when he teased me about a prison, that this would be his last meal.

"Okay, how do you want it cooked?"

"Rare, and I'll have fried potatoes with it," he said.

Gracious me, I thought. *He's up to something.*

"That'll take some time, so come down to the kitchen with me and you can watch your investment program, while I fix our dinner."

Finding something he liked to eat was becoming more difficult because he said food didn't have any taste, now. But the steak had all the taste he wanted.

He slowly chewed every small bite of his steak and literally drooled with delight. I took a mental picture to store in my heart. He ate a few bites of potatoes, which smelled scrumptious to me, but I didn't eat any because of the fat. Then, because the warmth felt soothing on his throat, he decided to focus on his Bushmills.

After I tucked George into bed that night, I sat by his side while he slept, looking around our exceptionally large master suite on the third floor of our townhouse. I knew how blessed we were to be so comfortable. The walls of our bedroom, windowed for more than thirty feet, looked onto magnificent bird-filled trees. We loved listening to the bird songs. His music system played constantly as he changed the programs from his bed with a special monitor. His computer was close by on his favorite antique desk, as he monitored his investments over the months. I kept fresh flowers on his desk that he thanked me for so often.

Early on, against his objection, I bought a large flat television screen so that he could watch his investment programs. "I don't want a television in our bedroom," he used to say. In no time, he was pleased to be able to watch his favorite financial commentators and programs. We watched the programs together so he could feel more confident in my capacity to manage our financial portfolio.

My twin bed was close by which gave him comfort. Only a week earlier, he had climbed into my bed after his dinner, when the nursing assistant had been caring for him. She tried to get him to go to his own bed. But he wouldn't get out of my bed.

When I came home, her eyes were huge as she explained to me what happened. I told her it was fine and not to worry. I didn't wake him. Instead, I slept in his bed, and was pleased to learn that his bed was more comfortable than mine.

Two hours later, while I was still reminiscing, George woke up. I heard him call, "Phyllis, why can't I get rid of this cold? I've got fish brushes in my stomach." The pharyngeal muscles in his throat were in spasm, and he couldn't stop coughing. I gave him a comfort dose of Ativan and put two drops of morphine under his tongue, which was swollen, gray and hard.

He slept quietly the rest of the night. I wondered if the fish brushes were his steak dancing in his tummy. That night he wet his bed, something he expected would happen when he was close to dying. This was a line he could not cross and consider it living.

On Tuesday, he refused any food, except sips of Ensure and water. Our hospice nurse, Joy, visited that day and noted that George's general appearance and reactions were considerably weaker. His blood pressure was low relative to his usual reading. He didn't remember her name even though she had been his nurse for many months. She suggested that I start the Ativan medicine if he showed any anxiousness.

With great glee, George told her about his steak dinner. She was surprised, looking at me to determine if he was teasing. He loved teasing her.

I told her about his steak feast, and that I had given him a low dose of Ativan when he started to become uncomfortable.

"Phyllis didn't get me up to go to the bathroom last night," he told her. "I can't use the commode. I have to go to the bathroom to pee."

She asked George if it would help him to have a condom catheter put on his penis so that he didn't wet his bed at night. It could be taken off during the day when he was up. "This is your decision. I won't put it on unless you agree," she said.

"If it will help Phyllis, put it on."

I went into the closet and wept. I knew we had crossed another threshold. He had made me promise from the beginning that he wouldn't have a urine bag hanging on his wheelchair like the people he had seen at the first ALS meeting. And yet, out of concern for me, he agreed to have such an arrangement. He'd worked so hard to be a partner with me in this adventure.

He'd frequently read Hank Dunn's book, *Hard Choices for Loving People*, and understood all the options he had to prepare for his death, a great private preparation for each of us. He understood that stopping fluids would not cause him to suffer.

But the catheter wouldn't stay on, so the nurse planned to come back the next day and put in an internal catheter. He said nothing. He had made his choice not to continue living when he refused any food, and little water. Because his body systems were so broken down, he had little reserve to nourish his body.

George had a line he clearly drew. When all systems weren't working, it was time to bail out of the airplane. And bail he did when he determined it was time, not when the disease determined this. George approached his life as an engineer since that was how he was trained. He was still in charge when he chose to die.

As I was washing his face with a cool face cloth that he always enjoyed, I remembered what he had told me a year ago that he had read somewhere: "We eat to live. We stop eating to die."

Neighbors and friends came to visit him that Tuesday evening. He was always up for his friends as he joked and swapped stories with them. He never lost his gentlemanly manner, or his social skills. He could fool people. He could use jokes and clichés of past life and everyone thought he was fine and not going to die. After they left, he asked me who they were and promptly fell asleep. We had crossed another threshold.

After George stopped eating and drinking Ensure, he spent his time resting quietly, sometimes with his eyes closed, sometimes listening to his music. He spoke very little and asked for nothing. But when I would ask him if he wanted water or ice chips in his mouth, he shook his head no, his mouth set in determination. When I asked him anything, he barely answered, turning his head from side to side.

On Wednesday, when I saw Anna giving him a shower, I knew this was his last shower. His body was rounded, his bones were prominent, and he was caved into his side towards the shower wall. I asked her to stop. After drying him and putting on his pajamas, I walked him back to bed.

George said, "Look. I'm still standing tall." His goal was to stand on his feet until the last day he was alive. He was proud of himself and boasted a wide smile. I hugged him and told him I knew he could do it.

"Thank you. Not without you, I couldn't," he said.

The hospice nurse returned later that morning and inserted the rubber catheter into George's penis, which turned into a long procedure. George's prostate gland had been enlarged since 1996 when he was treated for cancer of the prostate gland. Consequently the catheter drained bloody urine for a couple of hours while George rested. Apparently, it was painful to George to have the catheter in place.

"Take the damn thing out, Phyllis," he said. I called

Joy and she agreed that I should take it out. She knew I was a nurse. "You know how to do it, I'm sure." She added, "You'll have to put him in diapers so he doesn't develop bedsores."

I cut the small balloon of water that held the catheter in place, and removed it.

I remembered my promise to George not to put him in diapers. I knew his systems were nearly finished and he wasn't taking anything to drink except small sips of water. He was not likely to have a bowel movement since he hadn't eaten and his body was too weak to push anything out. He had little urine either.

"George, I bought some 'party pants' for you to wear in case you need to pee before I can help you. You can party all night and not get in trouble. These will keep your bed dry so you aren't uncomfortable."

"OK, Phyllis, let's have the party pants." He added, "Now where's the party." He smiled a gentle upturning of his lips that was almost like a kiss.

When I settled him in bed that night I asked, "Are there some sleeping positions that are more comfortable for you than others? I know you can't turn by yourself. Could you help me with this?"

"No, whatever you do is fine."

"I know that's not true since I'm not perfect, and I can't read your mind."

"When I'm unhappy, I'll let you know. But keep me sitting up."

At midnight I saw him become restless and try to turn himself. I helped him resettle, rubbed his back, and raised the bottom of his bed to keep him from sliding.

While I was concerned more with his immediate physical condition, George was more concerned with the spiritual. He had shown me the heavy metal Buddha statue he had kept in his airplane, and the many other statues he kept in his office and our bedroom. He observed many practices of the Buddhist tradition before and after we married. He practiced meditation daily and read his Buddhist teachings.

George wanted a peaceful, quiet death. He didn't need to tell people goodbye. Those he loved knew he loved them. Their presence wouldn't help him at all and would only be stressful. George believed that you do what is best for yourself at this time. He wasn't interested in resolutions, apologies, or other such rituals at death.

Unlike my experiences as a nurse working with dying patients in hospitals, I smelled the soft scent of roses around George when he was dying, not the odor of dead and decaying flesh. Also, George walked until the day he died and was never bed bound with his illness.

We sat in companionable silence for some time. It worked for us. Like many people, George was extremely tired as he was dying. He drifted in and out of sleep, as though he had crossed over to another world and didn't want to be summoned back to this one. I frequently changed the cool washcloth on his forehead. Sometimes, he grinned when I did it. He was peaceful even when his breathing changed and became irregular.

I listened to symphony music as I sat by his bed all evening and into early Thursday morning. Holding his hand at 3 a.m., I saw that his death was imminent. His breathing became sporadic, his skin changed rapidly from hot to cool, and his face became taut and pale. I told him that I loved him and he had my permission to do whatever he wanted. I was surprised when he looked up from his pillow and asked, "Am I home?"

I told him, "Yes, you're home. This is some fancy hotel for a nursing home." He grinned, as one corner of his mouth turned up. I wished him a good flight.

For me, this was an act of love, not an act of death. It was an act of letting go. I was freeing him to die, and he needed death at this time. He was stress-free, and relaxed. The best way for him to die was to have someone he loved simply be there. And not judge, or cry.

George didn't fear death, he just slid into it. He took his last breaths ten minutes later while I held his hand. The experience of death for him was silence. It seemed as though it happened in a blink. His death was still and mannerly, similar to the way he lived. To me his face had a noble cast as his facial features tightened into what looked like an aristocratic mask.

Our life together began and ended the same way. On July 10, 1970 he popped up on my doorstep for our blind date, and smiled at me. On March 20, 2003, he looked up from his pillow, for our last date, and smiled at me. Laughter and humor were our bonds in living and in dying. We walked this final journey together, alone. That was his wish. There was no big fanfare, no last hurrah. For him, it was a life well-lived and a death full of love.

Having a loved one with a fatal illness doesn't have to stop your life. You can still live life to the fullest, as we did. You can walk away when it is done, as I did, with an intact heart, because I survived one of life's most humbling experiences: taking the ultimate journey with someone I loved.

We were close to the end of our symphony. I had honored all his decisions except the last one: to leave his home standing tall.

MISSION ACCOMPLISHED

I have fought the good fight,
I have finished my course,
I have kept the faith.
II Timothy 4:7

After George died, I had no energy to move. I sat by his side and revisited some of the memories we had built during these last years. The ceiling fan buzzed above my head. The only other sound I heard was the heater when it cycled. Life had left the house.

Since I felt chilled, I ran the bath water especially hot, craving bubbles and the sweet scent of lavender. I sank into the tub and wept.

Suddenly, I remembered that seven close friends were coming to lunch at noon. I pondered whether I should cancel. I knew that George wouldn't have cancelled under any circumstances. I decided that their company would be comforting to me.

In a daze, I realized that I had to call the hospice nurse to come and officially pronounce George dead.

After she arrived and examined George, we reviewed the necessary hospice protocol for discharging him from their services, and the legal issues of declaring him dead, signing papers, and flushing down the toilet his unused narcotic and other medicines. I thanked the nurse for all the services that hospice so graciously provided us for over a year.

I waited another couple of hours and called the transport service to take George to the funeral home. On the telephone, I instructed the drivers to back their vehicle into our garage, which I would leave open for them to close. This way the neighbors wouldn't be disturbed with vehicles doing strange things during the night.

In the meantime, I called Dianne and Harvey who arrived shortly before the transport drivers. The drivers pulled their SUV into my garage, and then closed the garage door. I noted that the senior driver, who wore glasses, didn't resemble other funeral home drivers that I had seen. He wore a windbreaker and a lackluster shirt. The younger assistant wore nondescript casual clothes, and he appeared to be a trainee. He didn't know what to do with himself or his hands, which he stuffed into his pockets. His eyes were half closed during most of their visit.

"Hello, I'm Phyllis Langton and these are my friends Dianne and Harvey Kammerer." I stretched out my right hand to shake theirs. They introduced themselves, and offered weak, limp handshakes. My husband used to comment on people's handshakes, especially men's, and his comments weren't always nice. But I had just one mission on my mind, and that was to keep the promise I'd made to him. I was going to be sure he rode down the elevator as he left his home, standing tall.

After telling them where George's body was to be taken, the senior driver asked "Would you please take us to Mr. Thomas and tell us the best way to carry him out?" They were not robust men, and I imagined the thoughts that were going through his head. How much does Mr. Thomas weigh? Will he fit on the little stretcher we brought? What floor is he on—hopefully not the fourth? And how much work is it going to be to get him into the SUV?

"He's on the third floor," I answered. "We have an elevator, and I'd like him brought down in it. My husband wants to ride in the elevator one more time, standing up."

The men stared at me with wide-open eyes and blank faces. I waited, but they said nothing. So I told them my plan. "Please wrap Mr. Thomas securely so he stands in the elevator leaning against the wall with ties around his waist that are secured to the elevator wall railings. Leave his face uncovered so I can see him and talk to him during his last ride out of the house, and our last ride together in our physical bodies."

The senior driver's pale face began to show strain. He was middle-aged but didn't look any healthier than George had. Now he'd stuffed his hands into his pockets, too and began to shift his feet back and forth. "Mrs. Langton," he said, "we can't do that. It's too dangerous. He might fall."

I wanted to say: So what if he falls? He's dead. He can't hurt himself. But instead I said, "I'll wrap him myself."

"No, no. That just won't work. We've never been asked to do this before, and we don't know how to do what you're asking."

"Maybe we can work together," I said. "He won't fall if we wrap him carefully and then tie him to the handrail. Besides, I will be holding him during the entire ride. This was very important to my husband, who was a test pilot and fighter pilot in three wars. He wanted to accomplish his mission of leaving his home standing tall on his feet, instead of leaving feet first."

They nodded in what seemed to be agreement. We worked together.

Slowly we prepared George for his final ride. We reinforced the wrapping around him until it was firm enough to support him. The men lifted him to his feet and held him steady with their arms securely around him. We finished our work and walked him to the elevator. When he was standing and secure in the elevator, I asked Dianne and Harvey to escort the drivers to the bottom level where George and I would meet them. I closed the elevator door.

So that I could have more time with George than it took to travel three floors, I didn't push the button to start the elevator. I switched the light to 'on' so we could talk awhile before we began his last ride to the bottom floor, standing tall.

My own feelings were fuzzy since I was so mentally

and physically exhausted, but I focused on keeping my promise to him for his last ride. I remember talking and reminiscing with him about the many pictures I kept on the elevator walls for his enjoyment during our daily rides. Many were of our Ireland trip when I surprised him for his 73rd birthday. He had no idea where we were headed until we stood in line at Air Lingus Airline in Boston, and I handed him his ticket. "But, Phyllis," he said, "I have appointments."

"I know," I said. "I cancelled them."

The pictures of our daughter's wedding were still funny. Walking her down the aisle, she was so nervous, George had difficulty keeping her from running. When they arrived at the railing, George told Bishop Eastman, "Hurry up and marry them before she gets away and runs out of the church."

Close to his face were pictures of two of our darling granddaughters, Claire and Lorna, playing soccer. "Coach Edward," their father, had arranged a special game in George's honor after the May 2001 season was over. We drove to Nashville for the game, and his eyes filled with tears as five-year-old Claire made five goals against the boys: the game score was six-two. Claire was so excited and so proud of herself and her grandpa that she ran into him at full speed to hug him after the game. She grabbed his legs, and they both fell over, laughing all the way to the ground.

All these pictures broke my heart. We had shared our lives; we had shared George's death, as he unconditionally trusted me to make this journey with him. He had given me the gift of caring for him until he took his last breath.

Now he was in a distant place where I could no longer reach him. As we approached the ground floor, I thought I saw the weariness fade from his face. He was completing his mission. I didn't close his eyes when he died, and to me his eyes were sparkling. He had a smile on his face. As the elevator door opened on the ground floor, his blue eyes still twinkled at me. I will always remember him that way.

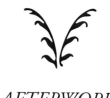

AFTERWORD

Books are the treasured wealth of the world and the inheritance of generations and nations.
Henry David Thoreau

For more than sixty years, I have been working in the 'field of dying.' Death and dying have been my constant *professional* companions. In 1964, as a nurse, medical sociologist and researcher, I published an article in *Nursing Forum*: "Attitudes Towards Death: An Emerging Mental Health Problem." The 'moral tone' has not changed since then. We continue to avoid facing our mortality, fearing death and dying. Comedian Woody Allen tells us, "I'm not afraid of death, I just don't want to be there when it happens."

In October 2000, when my husband was diagnosed with ALS, death and dying became my constant *personal* companions. I pondered, *how do I live with them?* My years of experience as a nurse working 8-10 hour shifts a day with dying patients did not prepare me for doing this 24/7 for 365 days a year. I wasn't sure I was up to the task. As always in my life, when I faced challenges, I began a journal. Putting my feelings on paper—whether real or not—exposed me to myself. Words helped me construct a world that made sense; a world that I could reside in without fear. Writing it down made life's events matter, and encouraged me to reflect, often changing my course of action. I found I was up to the task.

After a few weeks, I showed it to my husband who smiled and said, "Oh, my, you saw everything. I thought I had you fooled." In a humble, selfless voice he added, "You're always writing books. Maybe you should write one about us."

My life has been guided by the wisdom of F. Scott Fitzgerald who calls our attention to the difficulty of accepting the tension of opposites that we live with, while still retaining the ability to function. Writing the journal kept me aware of the opposite journeys we were travelling together: my husband's journey toward death, and my journey toward life. Writing showed me how to live in the spaces of these tensions, accept them and work to change our direction so we didn't become victims of ALS. By choosing to care for each other as partners to the end, our love grew to a far more intimate place than we could have imagined. Consequently, we were prepared to let go with humor, grace and high spirits.

Writing *Last Flight Out* was a comforting yet sometimes wrenching experience. I missed George's humor, his kindness, his intelligence and his company. There are some hurts that engrave the soul so deeply that we are forever changed. Yet, writing can provide boundaries to the pain. I found that writing what was inside of me lessened my grief by creating distance from the daily tasks of our exhausting journey. We were two ordinary folks, not celebrities, whose lives were blessed from the richness of family and friends.

We embraced life to its fullest by figuring out the rhythms of living with the constantly changing plateaus of a fatal illness. Without losing our sense of ourselves, we accepted kindnesses offered by a community of professionals and friends in pursuit of a peaceful quality of life and death at home. While there may be a limit to what medicine can cure, there is no limit to how much we can care.

Our grandchildren were touched deeply when they read the stories of their adventures caring for their grandpa. Stories amplify memories that can add to pictures in photo albums, thus giving meaning and depth to cross-generational connections. As they read their story, both girls smiled broadly and their eyes showed tender compassion. The younger child said, "I didn't realize that was the last time I would see Grandpa George. . . I can't wait to read this story to my children." My answer to her was: "Please wait."

After my husband died in 2003, I directed my energy into two major efforts. The first was to help families with ALS and educate the public about ALS. Consequently, I served as Executive Secretary on the DC/MD/VA ALS board for four years and worked with ALS patients and families in their homes, which I continue to do today. My second effort was to write the book my husband requested: an awesome task.

As a social scientist and researcher, I had no idea how to write a memoir. Thus I started by attending classes at the University of Iowa during the summer programs, the Writer's Center in Bethesda all year, online classes with Writer's Digest, and joining two writing groups. With encouragement from peers, I applied to the Hambidge Center for the Creative Arts in Georgia for a fellowship in the Artists Residency program. I was accepted. Repeat residencies there were followed by fellowships at the Ragdale Foundation, and the Robert M. MacNamara Foundation.

While at the Hambidge Center, I was fortunate to meet Heather Tosteson, a fiction writer and poet and co-publisher, with Charles Brockett, of Wising Up Press. Through their encouragement, I published four chapters of this book in separate anthologies, listed in the Acknowledgments section of this book, and co-edited an anthology, *View from the Bed, View From the Bedside.*

During this period, I was invited to join the Writers Collective of Wising Up Press. I have been enriched many times over from the close association of this Collective as we work together through retreats, read others' work, and share vibrant conversations inside and outside our Collective about the larger social justice issues surrounding us in this fast world. In the Collective, I have found a sense of usefulness to my community, small and large. For me, a true measure of my life is how useful I am to my community.

After a lifetime of writing scholarly works for my colleagues who are more comfortable with facts and data,

I am following my passion with words, writing another memoir. *Sweet Abandon* is the story of my search for family after being born in a Salvation Army home in Boston during the Great Depression and being left there by my mother.

ACKNOWLEDGMENTS

With this book I give a special thanks to my family and all our friends for their endless contributions to our lives before and during our journey. Thank you for listening to me for several years discuss this book and for offering critical suggestions. My heartfelt thanks to all of you. I thank my daughter Phyleen for contributing to the title.

Artist Residency Fellowships from the Hambidge Center for the Creative Arts, Robert M. MacNamara Foundation, and the Ragdale Foundation made it possible for me to work uninterrupted and to associate with many fine artists from a variety of genres. These opportunities changed my life by creating lasting friendships that renewed my confidence to enjoy my remaining life with words.

Many thanks to Joan Hammel, well-known singer and songwriter, for taking the picture on the book cover while we were residents at the MacNamara Foundation, Westport Island, Maine.

Thank you Karen Mortenson for your fine editing early on; Jill Breckenridge for excellent editing in the middle; and finally Heather Tosteson's vision in turning this story into a book. Her talents are extraordinary.

Four chapters in *Last Flight Out: Living, Loving & Leaving* appeared in slightly different form in the following Wising Up anthologies: "Mission Accomplished" in *Illness & Grace: Terror & Transformation*; "Waiting" and "Celebrating Life is Forever" in *Love After 70*; and "Dying at Home" in *View from the Bed: View from the Bedside.*

Lastly, my deep gratitude goes to my husband, George Thomas, who was a full-time partner with me throughout this journey. By choosing to share the care, our love grew to a more intimate place than could be imagined.

DISCUSSION GUIDE

Through the intimacy of reading the pleasures and sorrows that were part of our journey, I hope you, the reader, will find *LAST FLIGHT OUT* to be a living and dying *friendly* book. My wish is to spark conversations that will bring us together to discuss these topics so we can prepare proactively.

SIX MONTHS

*After George was diagnosed with Lou Gehrig's disease (ALS),
his doctor told him he probably had six months to live and
to go out and do all the things he had postponed doing. In
addition, he prescribed an experimental drug, Rilutek, that
had the potential to increase his life a month or two. George
refused to take the drug because of the potential serious side
effects that might reduce his current quality of life.*

1. Try to imagine what it would be like to be told by your
doctor that you probably have six months to live. How
would you process that message? Do you think doctors
should tell patients that information if they don't ask for
it? If you only had a limited time to live, how would you
live it?

2. Would you share the news with your family and friends?
Why or why not? When and how would you do this while
still protecting your own privacy and personal rights?

3. Would you consider taking an experimental drug if it
might increase your life another month or two, but had
the potential to reduce the quality of your life? Would
your decision be different if you were younger—or had
dependants? Do you think patients in these circumstances
should feel an obligation to participate in experimental
protocols that may have long-term benefits for others?
Explain.

4. Describe your reaction to George's statement after he heard the bad news, "I know what's going to be on my death certificate. That's more than you can say?" Were you surprised?

LOOKING FORWARD

We aren't comfortable talking about death and dying but these topics are always there. Why is it hard to have these conversations? To live well with a fatal illness, we need to know the quality of life and death we want and how to negotiate these wishes with our families, or whomever we have entrusted to make these decisions.

1. Describe your own situation at this time in terms of preparing for living and dying in the event of a fatal illness, or if a tragic event would happen that left you unable to care for yourself. Have you designated someone who will take care of you and make decisions for you? Do you think such a plan is necessary? Where do you prefer to die: at home, in a hospital, or another place?

2. Have you decided the specific kind of medical care you want or don't want, such as resuscitation (CPR), artificial feeding, ventilator (breathing machine), and other options to keep you alive? Have you discussed this with your doctor?

3. Describe your experiences in caring for someone who trusted you to carry out their life and dying decisions. Did you encounter any conflicts when acting in this capacity? If so, how were these resolved?

4. Have you or someone you know experienced a situation where someone has not made their wishes known and disputes arose among family members? Can you imagine some of the conflicts that could exist in such a situation?

TALKING ABOUT DEATH WITH YOUR DOCTOR

When George had lived a year after he was told he probably had six months to live, we visited his doctor to share his medical directive. We asked for his agreement to honor his medical directive that stated no CPR, no ventilator or other means to keep him alive and to die peacefully at home. His doctor was reluctant to agree with this directive because he was his 'treating' physician. Again, he asked him to take the drug, Rilutek. Again, George declined.

1. Do you think a physician should be reluctant to provide care for a terminal patient who doesn't follow his orders to take a drug with potential severe side effects? If a patient wants to enter Hospice Care, they need a referral from their physician. Do physicians have an obligation to refer a patient to another physician who will accept the patient's medical directives?

2. How do patients with fatal illnesses find doctors who are willing to care for them when they disagree with some treatment regimes and end-of-life care plans?

RITUALS AND THEIR SIGNIFICANCE

Americans are widely known to embrace rituals including cultural ones like Halloween, religious ones like Christmas, and familial ones like weddings, birthdays and more. Rituals help bring order to a chaotic unpredictable world, connecting us with others and reinforcing our identity. Many people feel it is important in the circumstances of a fatal disease to continue celebrating rituals and possibly create new ones. We created new rituals: celebrating his birthday each year on the same day he was diagnosed with ALS and told he had six months to live.

1. What rituals are important to you? Would you make these a continuing part of your life if you were diagnosed with a terminal illness?

2. We laugh hardest when we laugh with others. What are some ways we can bring humor into the illness situation without being disrespectful? Do you think that humor is important in keeping tragedy from having the last word?

3. Have you observed other people developing new rituals during a fatal illness? Describe what you saw and its effects.

FINDING AND ACCEPTING HELP

As the disease ravaged George's body, we faced many challenges that required us to change our direction. At first, I tried to do it all, almost in a manic sense. Then the exhaustion set in as I began to make mistakes that could have been harmful to us. I had to step back, find and accept help. This was a problem because we valued our privacy and independence. He didn't want strangers in our home caring for him when I needed to be away, but he couldn't be left alone. To learn ways to work on this, we joined the ALS local chapter support groups for patients and families. In addition, I attended the support groups for ALS caregivers only. I also contacted a private agency and employed several nursing assistants. This latter effort was a constant struggle and emotional roller coaster ride for both of us, ending in disaster. When friends continued to call and ask, "What can we do?" I organized a plan so that when they called, I had a task for them. We learned to accept help from our many friends.

1. Describe your experiences with support groups of any kind and how these were helpful, or not.

2. What have been your experiences with employing nursing assistants from private agencies?

3. What others ways would you find and accept help if you were the primary caregiver?

4. Denial is an important coping mechanism in illness, especially progressive illness, but it can also add more stress to the caregiver as George's reluctance to use a wheelchair did. What balance must caregivers strike between the patient's desire to preserve his or her independence, or appearance of independence, and the cost of that choice to the caregiver? Would you have made the same choices that I did? Acted sooner? Later?

ANGELS OF LIFE

Relationships change as the illness progresses. We decided to enter the hospice care at home program early. George told the nurse he felt hospice care would improve his quality of life and death so that he didn't become a burden to me. Consequently, more people became regular visitors to our home: nursing aides to help with bathing and dressing several mornings a week, as well as bi-weekly visits by a nurse and monthly visits by a physician. When our friends heard we had entered hospice care at home, many assumed he was dying immediately and stopped calling. In our case, we were in hospice care for over a year.

1. What is your knowledge of and experience with hospice care?

2. Have you known anyone who has died at home or in a hospital with hospice care?

3. Would you consider hospice care an option when you prepare your plan for living and dying with a fatal illness? Why or why not?

NURTURE YOURSELF

As we continue to live longer with many diseases that require individual care, we will all experience the need to provide or receive care. When you are responsible for caring for someone for an extended period, it is important that you find time for positive, nurturing interactions with others, outside the sickness environment so you don't become a victim of the disease. Without this space you may lack the strength to deal with all of the emotions you experience, including guilt and anger—anger at the disease and circumstances, not the patient. In his typical flyboy humor, George would tell me: "Go out and have a good time, but don't pick up any men because I'm not dead yet." When I went out, I had his friends visit and keep him out of mischief. Nurturing yourself prevents you from becoming sucked in by the disease.

1. Have you or others you have known been the primary person responsible for providing care for someone over an extended period of time? Describe your experiences or the experiences of others that you have observed.

2. Can you imagine ways to help caregivers find time for their own positive, nurturing interactions with others?

3. We really don't know how much we can do until we do it. Have you ever pushed yourself beyond what you thought you could and should do? Describe this experience and how you moved out of the situation to nurture yourself.

A PLACE FOR CHILDREN

We protect young children from participating in death and illness events. More people die in hospitals and nursing homes today than in their homes. Hospitals haven't encouraged visiting privileges for children in intensive care units where many patients die. When children participate with their families caring for a dying relative, they feel useful and less afraid of the mystery of death. George's grandchildren shared their love with him by feeding him, washing him and other exciting tasks. They gave him the benefit of their wisdom for living.

1. Do you think children should be included in helping to care for a dying relative? What has been your experience with children caring for dying family members?

2. How would you prepare a child for what she will hear or see, for example, the condition of the patient, and any equipment to make the patient comfortable?

3. Did you experience anyone among your family or close friends dying during your childhood? Describe how your family included you, or excluded you in this process. Was death talked about in your family in such a way that you were included in the conversation or allowed to participate? What effect has this had on how you view death and dying?

LETTING GO

In the chapter "Down but Not Out," George lost consciousness and stopped breathing for a prolonged period. I didn't call 911 because he had made me promise there would be no heroic measures to save his life, and that he would die at home. Later, when he recovered to tell the story to his friends, they were shocked and dismayed that I would let him die in the elevator, rather than take him to the emergency room. Hank Dunn, chaplain in nursing homes and hospice for over seventeen years, writes in <u>Hard Choices for Loving People</u> that fatal isn't the worst outcome for dying people. From his experience and research he concludes that the real struggles for families "letting go" are emotional and spiritual, not medical, legal, ethical or moral aspects of the decision process.

1. Identify and discuss some emotional and spiritual issues that might affect how families make decisions to keep their loved ones living with artificial measures when they may actually have a need for death.

2. Have you experienced any such situations yourself when caring for someone who was dying? If so, how did you work this out with other family members?

3. Often one family member objects to letting a person die, even when it is the dying person's wish. What resources can be made available to help families resolve these choices in the direction of always granting patients' wishes?

DYING AT HOME

According to William Colby in his book, <u>Unplugged: Reclaiming Our Right to Die in America</u>, eighty percent of Americans die in some type of institution, rather than at home. Yet surveys show that most cancer patients in the United States express a preference to die at home.

1. What factors do you think might explain the discrepancy between what people say they prefer and what they experience?

2. What are some ways we can ensure that patients' wishes are promoted and protected so they die at home even if the family doesn't accept their decision?

3. Describe your ideas of a peaceful death. Talk about where you prefer to be when you die and why. Can you think of any reasons why your wishes may not be carried out?

4. Do you know anyone who has died at home? Did you feel that the person should have been taken to the hospital? Have you been present when someone has died at home?

SAYING GOODBYE

Saying goodbye to our families and friends is a common death ritual of some religions and cultures. However, such rituals may hinder an individual from following different cultural practices that put as paramount the wishes of the dying person. George did not want to say a special goodbye when he was dying or to have people around observing him die. He had already said goodbye some time ago to those he loved and respected. As part of his private Buddhist practice and preparation for death, he needed to be conscious, sitting up, and stress free when he was ready to let go, with me holding his hand.

1. What was your reaction when George wanted to die quietly at home with no one present except his wife because it would create less stress for him?

2. Do you think the dying person's wishes should have priority over the living in this situation?

3. Can you imagine any circumstances where family members' wishes have priority over the dying persons' wishes of being present at the death of a family member? Have you experienced or observed any family conflicts in this area?

4. If someone you know dies tragically or unexpectedly, would it be important to you to find ways to say farewell?

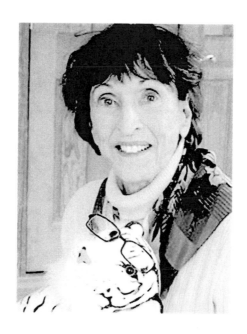

PHYLLIS A. LANGTON, Ph.D., R.N., Professor Emerita, Sociology, George Washington University, is the author of more than twenty-five articles and books. Her last textbook was published in 2005. She holds a Ph.D. from UCLA and an active registered nurse license from California for over fifty-five years. She has taught Sociology of Health and Illness (including Death and Dying) for over forty years. Her interest in creative non-fiction writing began in 2000 when her husband was diagnosed with Lou Gehrig's disease (ALS) and given six months to live. She served four years as Secretary of DC/MD/VA ALS Board to educate the public and support families with ALS. She is currently working on a second memoir, *Sweet Abandon,* about her search for family. She lives in McLean, Virginia. You can learn more about her at www.phyllisalangton.com.

CPSIA information can be obtained at www.ICGtesting.com
Printed in the USA
BVOW011659131111

275971BV00001B/23/P